THE SCIENTIST WHO WASN'T THERE

ABOUT THE AUTHOR

Joanne's debut book, *The Scientist Who Wasn't There*, was awarded the first Bridport Prize for Memoir. She was a barrister for many years and has continued to work in other legal roles, in a career spanning nearly four decades. She lives in Sussex.

THE SCIENTIST WHO WASN'T THERE

A TRUE STORY OF STAGGERING DECEPTION

JOANNE BRIGGS

ITHAKA

First published in the UK by Ithaka Press
An imprint of Bonnier Books UK
5th Floor, HYLO, 105 Bunhill Row,
London, EC1Y 8LZ

Hardback ISBN: 978-1-80418-972-6
Trade Paperback ISBN: 978-1-80418-973-3
Ebook ISBN: 978-1-80418-974-0
Audiobook ISBN: 978-1-80418-975-7

A CIP catalogue record for this book is available from
the British Library.

Typeset by IDSUK (Data Connection) Ltd

Printed and bound in Great Britain by Clays Ltd, Elcograf S.p.A

1 3 5 7 9 10 8 6 4 2

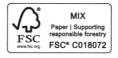

The authorised representative in the EEA is
Bonnier Books UK (Ireland) Limited.
Registered office address: Floor 3, Block 3, Miesian Plaza,
Dublin 2, D02 Y754, Ireland
compliance@bonnierbooks.ie
www.bonnierbooks.co.uk

To Mike, James and Luke,
for being there

CONTENTS

AUTHOR'S NOTE

A few words about whether this is 'a true story'.

I'm not an investigative journalist or a scientist, and I can only talk about my own perspective on Primodos, which is related to the story I wanted to tell, about my dad. If you want to know about Primodos, go to reputable sources, read everything you can about it from all sides, then decide for yourself what you think is right.

The language used in this book to describe the drug Primodos mirrors that of the report of the All-Party Parliamentary Group for Hormone Pregnancy Tests, *A Bitter Pill: Primodos – The Forgotten Thalidomide*, published in February 2024. It is acknowledged that Bayer Schering does not accept that there is a causal link between Primodos and birth defects.

I'm also not a historian: what I've written is a memoir, not a historical account. I think memory is to memoir what truth is to authenticity, so you can't have the latter without the former, but there's a lot more to it than that. My memory of the past is as much made up of dreams, impressions, false beliefs, fantasies, feelings and notions as it is of facts, and it's this whole experience of the past – my past – viewed from the present, which I hope makes my memoir authentic. But is that a true story? Well, yes, it is to me, and I hope it tells my truth to you. If you'd been there at the time, of course, you might have seen it differently.

PROLOGUE

Somewhere, there's nine minutes of my dad preserved on film, though I've never seen it. It's been a long time since I last saw my dad alive, moving and talking, so I'd like to be able to watch him again, if only on a screen. But though I know it's somewhere – the whole thing even has a catalogue number in the British Film Institute archive – it seems I'm unlikely to get the chance.

It's part of a documentary called the *The Primodos Affair*, about a chemical substance that quite a few people believe changed their lives for the worse. The programme was made in 1980 by Thames Television but, thanks to a decades-old court order, it was never broadcast and is kept under lock and key to this day. Or, at least, I imagine it is. The film's physical whereabouts aren't very clear.

In my life, I've encountered many different versions of my dad, and two or three since he died in 1986. They confuse my memory, adding new shapes and colours to what I thought about him when I was a child, then a young person, and then different again, before his death when I was twenty-three. Sometimes a muddle, sometimes a pattern, like the rotations of a kaleidoscope.

When I was small, I believed my dad to be the only man who knew all science. After he left for a different life in another country, I had to explain his absence and defend myself against those who looked on me with pity, so I told them this was the reason why he wasn't there. I'd say: 'Although you think it is, my situation isn't sad at all. Because my dad isn't gone, he's just somewhere else, being a very famous scientist. He knows everything about outer space. And deadly poisons. And rare diseases. And having babies. Anything you can think of, really, he's an expert in it. He's a doctor and he's written hundreds and hundreds of brilliant books.'

To be fair to me, this wasn't childish ignorance and wishful thinking. Professor Michael Briggs seemed that way to a lot of other people as well. He appeared to be a man who had been everywhere, becoming an expert in everything in the process. He was a NASA space scientist turned pharmacologist, a renowned specialist in biochemistry, an adviser to the World Health Organization, and a university Dean of Sciences. He'd also written a stack of papers about the many things that interested him, from synthetic human hormones to meteorites and intergalactic travel. My dad used to talk with the same relaxed authority about time machines and alien lifeforms as he did about the more familiar frontiers of human knowledge, in a way that made all the things he said seem equally likely to be true.

Viewed from this angle, my dad was a twentieth-century phenomenon; this Michael Briggs was a self-made man and a modern hybrid. His own father had been an unskilled typewriter mechanic, so his roots were firmly in the working class. He'd started out with nothing besides his ambition and he had to make his own way in the scientific world. Which he did by taking chances. He moved between countries and continents, jumping from one opportunity to the next, surfing the waves of the post-war technology boom and grabbing hold of everything the Jet Age had to offer.

It was an era when there seemed to be no boundaries to scientific imagination, and no limits to what a man might become, if he wanted it enough.

Jump off cliffs, as science fiction writer Ray Bradbury said, and build your wings on the way down.

It didn't end well, unfortunately. You could say that the extent of my dad's ambition proved to be his undoing.

Just before my dad's sudden, somewhat mysterious death in 1986, a front-page feature in the *Sunday Times* accused this high-profile scientist of fabricating his research. What the article didn't mention – because then, very few people knew – was his involvement in the unresolved saga of Primodos. When the Primodos story resurfaced in 2020, it revealed one more variant of my dad but, more importantly, it uncovered the fragile and imperfect structure which had been hidden beneath them all. That was when I went in search of the man he really was.

I've wondered many times since what I would be now if I hadn't. If I'd allowed myself to carry on with the rest of my life in ignorance. Although, then again, sooner or later, isn't it the fate of every parent to be found out by their children, as considerably less than they'd pretended?

My brother always says the past doesn't exist, anyway. History and heritage are no more use to the living than fairy stories. It doesn't really matter if the priceless Old Master that was passed down with great reverence from the previous generation is actually nothing but a cheap fake in an old frame. Or if, on closer inspection, Grandma's twenty-carat tiara turns out to be paste.

Or even if the world's greatest scientist, who I once looked up to so much, wasn't really there at all.

PART 1

THE MAN WHO KNEW ALL SCIENCE

'. . . how much happier that man is who believes his native town to be the world, than he who aspires to become greater than his nature will allow.'

Victor Frankenstein,
Frankenstein by Mary Shelley

1

My dad was unexpectedly back in the papers in the summer of 2020, after a gap of many years. Halfway down an inside page, there was his familiar gaze and wry smile, in a publicity-style headshot. His picture was next to a feature about a pharmaceutical substance, which, like him, was gone and all but forgotten. The drug in question, Primodos, had its own stock photo, showing two small white pills in blisters on a plastic card.

A longer article with a bigger headline described how three quite different pharmaceutical inventions had been bundled together in an investigation, the Independent Medicines and Medical Devices Review, and a report of its conclusions had just been published. Problems with these three different things primarily affected women, and a woman had been chosen by Theresa May, a female prime minister, to advise her if anything should be done about them.

One of these medical products was much more familiar to me than the others: sodium valproate, a drug often prescribed to treat mood instability. I'm involved with the legal side of the detention and discharge of psychiatric patients, so because of the job I do I know that sodium valproate should not be given to pregnant women, due to the risk of birth defects. I've never knowingly met anyone affected by the second substance, pelvic mesh, although I'm aware it's used in surgical interventions for various conditions and could go calamitously wrong.

The third, Primodos, a synthetic hormone pregnancy test, I'd never heard of at all, at the time.

Synthetic hormones of the kind that Primodos was made of had been one of my dad's many areas of interest, so it wasn't difficult to imagine how he might be mixed up with such a thing. But that was a very long time ago. And anyway, Primodos had not been on the market since 1978, so the article said.

Why bring it up now?

It seemed that a group of parents, all now old enough to be grandparents, together with some of their children, who were in mid- to late-middle age, were still waiting for their legal claims about Primodos to be heard by a court. They believed that the pregnancy test, given to them by doctors, had caused life-altering birth defects. Their cases had originally started in 1980, half a lifetime ago.

They've waited a very long time, I thought to myself. Probably too long, if my dad was in some way to blame.

The picture in the paper must have been taken some time in the early 1980s and was an unfortunate choice, given the context. His round face and his cheerful expression jarred with the subject under discussion, making him appear uninterested and uncaring. In a larger picture, Baroness Cumberlege, the chair of the inquiry, looked contrastingly thoughtful and stern. She'd said that, where harm had been caused by Primodos, the people affected should be given an apology and offered compensation.

I hadn't looked at a picture of my dad for many years and I realised that I was already several years older than he had ever been. He died in November 1986, when he was fifty-one and I was twenty-three, leaving behind barely a trace of himself. My brother looks a little more like him, as the years have gone by. I probably do, too. We have a few of his old books and some family photos. But there's really nothing much left of him. Apart from us, of course.

Even before the final breakdown of my parents' marriage in 1970, I remember my dad as being enigmatically absent. By that I mean he was typically somewhere else, with little evidence at the time or since to suggest where that might have been. In the 1960s and 70s, he was quite successful, as scientists go, so it was more than likely it was something to do with that. But to me, he was nearly always just out of reach. A constant presence on the periphery of my vision, who disappeared when I turned to face him.

The picture had set off a train of thought and a few hours later, I found myself in the loft, looking for my late mother's photo album. After our mother, Marion, had died, I'd persuaded my brother that he had more storage space than I did and, having assured him that I would return within the month to sort out the rest of her stuff, I'd left with an assortment of her belongings in a single cardboard box. The box was still where I'd left it when I'd pushed it up the ladder five years before, sitting on the rafters under the eaves.

The album was in among a collection of other things which I knew my mother valued rather more. A bundle of unfinished charcoal sketches rolled up in a perished elastic band; a clay maquette of a cross-legged female nude; a box of broken oil crayons; crystals with healing powers; a travelling watercolour paintbox and a folding easel; a bag of old foreign coins; some beach pebbles with holes in them threaded onto a piece of rick-rack braid.

I pulled out the album and wiped my sleeve over the padded leatherette cover. Inside, there were a lot of pictures of my brother and me, standing in front of highly patterned curtains or artificial Christmas trees in unremembered mid-century living rooms or playing side by side on concrete patios. But I'd never noticed before that, as time went on, there were fewer and fewer photographs. Gaps had been left unfilled, as neatly glued, densely packed collages of family celebrations gave way to sparser, higgledy-piggledy arrangements of random snaps. About halfway through the album, in the summer of 1969, the pictures ran out completely: after that, there was nothing but page after page of empty black sugar-paper. It was as if time had suddenly come to an end. Which in a way, it had.

My dad is there occasionally before the blank pages start, but only in sequences taken on family holidays in one Spanish resort or another. I know we are in Arenal d'en Castell, or Torremolinos, or Alcaufar, or Lloret de Mar, because my mother has written the name of the place on the picture's straight white edge, in blue ball-point pen. But the photos themselves are pretty much the same. My dad is always dressed in a dark blazer, pressed slacks and a tie, with a handkerchief visible in his top pocket, and the second button of his jacket permanently fastened. His aviator sunglasses make his facial expression hard to interpret, and in one of these pictures I look like a little girl holding hands with an operative from MI5, after he'd been issued with a wife and child as part of an elaborate plan to conceal his identity.

There are hardly any pictures of my mother, but in the days when pictures were taken with mechanical cameras on chemical film, one parent's absence from the family album wasn't necessarily

6

sinister. My mother's natural eye for the small details of ordinary life made her a good candidate to be the photographer who rarely appeared in front of the lens. But my dad's absence from nearly all our family photos was explicable only because he wasn't there to be photographed. The combined effect is that, if the album alone was to be believed, my brother and I barely had parents at all.

Turning over the last of the pictures in which my dad appears, I wondered when it was that my mother had realised the end was coming. Even in these short breaks from his customary absence, my dad was already leaving her, by stages. She seemed to be trying to capture this elusive husband and father on film, for posterity, so we might at least know what he'd once looked like. She even managed to get one last picture of them together. I imagined the moment when my mother handed the camera to a passing stranger, then reversed into position while explaining how it worked. The picture bears witness to the fact, if anyone ever doubted it, that they were once somewhere at the same time acting as parents, at least for the fraction of a second it took for the shutter to snap open and shut.

From then on, in his absence, the holiday images have an anxious atmosphere. My brother looks sideways out of the frame, away from an upturned fishing boat or a game of crazy golf, as if wondering where our dad had gone. These last few shots tell the story of an unseen woman, photographing her children as they were all about to be tipped into the unknown.

I hadn't been aware of how long I'd been in the attic until I noticed that below me, at the bottom of the ladder, the hallway was now in darkness. Before I put the album away, I flicked backwards through the pages, making my brother and me gradually reappear once more. It's like a cinematic device in a fantasy film, when time travellers have interfered with the past, upsetting the stability of the present. Family photographs begin to disintegrate, their essence suddenly conditional upon things that might never have happened at all.

2

My brother isn't very interested in human interest stories. When I call him later, he isn't aware our dad has become topical again, after thirty-odd years out of the limelight.

'So what's he done this time?' he says. 'Same old thing, I suppose?'

Two months before our dad's sudden death, a scandal about his scientific research had become international news. In September 1986, the *Sunday Times* ran a full-page close-up of his face with 'EXPOSED' written across it, as part of an exclusive under the headline 'The Bogus Work of Professor Briggs'.

'Oddly enough, it's not the fake research. Not this time. It's about something I've never heard of before. It must have happened about twenty years earlier, in the 1960s. Have you ever heard of Primodos?'

'Nope,' my brother replies. 'Why – should I have done?'

'It's a hormone pregnancy test, or rather it was, in tablet form. It was made by Schering Pharmaceuticals. There's a court case about it.'

'Ah, well, I've heard of them, obviously. Schering was where Dad was working, when we were kids. But how can a court case go on for half a century?'

My brother was born two years before me, in April 1961. He was the first child of a young couple on the move, who had stopped for a while in New Zealand. By the time I arrived, they were back in England and the cracks in family life were begin-ning to show. My brother is a more reliable witness about what happened to us as children than I am. He prefers to see it all as darkly funny, rather than painful or frightening.

'What can you really remember, from when we were young? I mean before 1970, when Dad was still there?'

'Not a lot,' my brother says. 'I suppose it would depend on what had made me think about it in the first place. Something I've seen before maybe, like a place or an object. Or musing about things you don't see anymore.'

'Like what?'

'Sticklebacks. Iron filings. Lunar landings. He and I had similar interests when I was young, so that kind of thing. But there's hardly anything specifically about Dad himself, to be honest. I remember when I was eight, he told me not to make chemical explosions in the shed unless I kept notes, like a proper scientist. Which was ironic, given what he was up to.'

'What about after he left?'

'After he'd gone, I think a lot of people felt sorry for us. Two little kids with no dad. It was a much more unusual thing in those days. I remember somebody saying we were from a "broken home" and wondering if the house was about to fall down.'

'I still can't bear it, if someone feels sorry for me,' I say. 'If anybody asked me where my dad was in those days, I'd tell them: "I don't see my daddy very much, but that's only because he lives in other countries. And before you say that's sad, it really isn't sad at all. I'm sure I'll see him very soon, when he goes to the World Health Organization in Geneva, or talks at an important conference, or invents a new kind of contraceptive pill, or something like that."'

'You did have a precocious talent for rhetoric, when small,' my brother says.

'It wasn't exaggeration, though, was it? That was our story. That was our life. Nobody outside the family had ever seen Dad, of course, what with all the moving around, so the other kids probably thought I was making it all up. When I said my dad's a scientist who's famous all around the world, who knows everything, they probably thought I was lying. But it was true, wasn't it?'

'Well, so we were led to believe,' my brother says.

3

When my dad turned fifty in August of 1985, he had a little over a year left to live. I don't specifically remember my dad's fiftieth birthday because I wasn't there. It wasn't a memorable day for me and, as far as I knew, he was ten thousand miles away. His birthdays had never been an event for the discarded skin of his family that he'd shed fifteen years before. I might have remembered to send him a card, though, to be honest, I very much doubt that I did.

When I turned fifty in 2013, he obviously wasn't there either, because he'd been dead for twenty-seven years. But for some of the time he'd been gone, I half-expected I'd see him again. This was a lasting side effect of something said by a journalist after the news broke that my dad was dead, that this turn of events was a bit too convenient to be true, given all the trouble he was in. I wasn't there when my dad died, of course. He was apparently dead and buried before I knew anything about it, far away, in another country. If I'd had some evidence, if I'd seen it with my own eyes, I'd have found it easier to believe. That's probably why my dad's unannounced reappearance became an impossible possibility for me, which took a long time to go away. But by the time I turned fifty, I was able to accept reality. At least, most of the time, and despite his last absence being his most enigmatic.

There's an alternative version of my fiftieth birthday in which there's a knock on the door and when I open it, my dad is standing there. He's smiling apologetically, having had no time to buy me a gift. I've rehearsed this scene both with and without a gift, and with gifts of various kinds, but I much prefer it without one.

Anyway.

Anyway, back in 1985, my dad had been a professor at an Australian university for nine years, which was more than double his previous record for staying in one place. My parents had met in Liverpool in 1957, when my mother was working in a dress factory and my dad was studying for a teaching diploma. Not long after their first date at a screening of the science fiction film *The Incredible Shrinking Man*, they set off for Canada. They were married in Montreal, then they moved to New York State. My brother was born in Upper Hutt, New Zealand before another move back to the USA, the West Coast this time.

My mother was eight months pregnant with me when my parents arrived back in England from Pasadena, in the autumn of 1963. After that, my dad had a job in the West Country, near Chippenham, which I'd always thought was something to do with animal feed. When he changed jobs again in 1966 and became research director of the pharmaceutical manufacturer Schering, we all moved about 150 miles east, from Wiltshire to Sussex. I was then three years old.

The Schering chapter also ended abruptly, but this time there was an additional cause for a sudden change of direction. In 1970, my dad left both my mother and the United Kingdom for another country, Zambia, and another relationship. He had met a woman at work who looked remarkably like my mother and not unlike his own: all three were small and slight, with boyishly close-cropped hair. He obviously went for a type.

He had two further jobs in two different countries, on two different continents. Then, in 1976, he was offered a senior professorship, at Deakin University in the Australian state of Victoria.

My dad should have spent his fiftieth birthday celebrating his newly acquired taste for steadiness and conformity, thinking about what new challenges his second half-century might hold for him. He could have reflected on some of the choices he was less proud of, and even wondered what he could do to build bridges and make amends. He could have opened a birthday card from me. But he didn't do any of that. Because, in August 1985, my dad made a sudden disappearance. He liquidated his assets, left his job and packed his bags. Then he slid out of Australia and was gone.

What happened in the 1980s at Deakin University is still a well-known case study in scientific fraud, although I've read that some of his colleagues at the time wanted to excuse my dad's behaviour on the grounds that he couldn't at the time have been in his right mind. These were probably people who'd become so invested in his backstory and his reputation that they couldn't believe what they were hearing. He was also capable of great personal charm, particularly when he wanted something. But for whatever reason, I think they fundamentally misunderstood what my dad's right mind was really like.

Deakin was the state of Victoria's newest university when my dad was chosen as its first dean of sciences in 1976, although it was at the time still under construction. Unlike many academic institutions, Deakin had not evolved naturally but was being created by amalgamating an existing teacher training college and an institute of technology, where my dad had briefly taken a job teaching science. Deakin was in some ways an experiment, as it was a regional university rather than city-based, and it was intended to support large numbers of distance-learners. An area of scrub in Waurn Ponds near Geelong had been chosen to become the university campus, a place crisscrossed with seasonal creeks and fallen gum trees that resembled a fantasy Martian desert on the cover of a paperback novel. But then building work began, and futuristic buildings, boulevards and plazas sprang up all over the barren landscape, driving out the drought-adapted amphibians and dust-bowl snakes that lived there into bushland beyond the new perimeter fence. Deakin finally opened its doors to students for its first trimester in 1977. As lectures began, there was a lot of enthusiasm on display, but rather less in the way of direct experience of specialist graduate education or research.

Deakin's first vice chancellor, Dr Fred Jevons, was a biochemist like my dad. They'd visited the science blocks as they were being built and Jevons believed they shared an ambitious vision for the department. He may well have ensured that very few questions were asked before my dad was offered the job. In particular, why someone so apparently successful wanted to work in a place like this, rather than going to a prestigious university in one of the world's great cities, with a well-established track record in the kind of thing he was interested in.

My dad's appointment was truly a coup for the new university. His CV boasted an Ivy League doctoral degree from Cornell, then a Doctor of Science degree, in recognition of his exceptional contribution to science by the age of only twenty-seven. He'd been a member of the elite space science research team at the NASA Caltech Jet Propulsion Laboratories in Pasadena, advising on biochemical aspects of manned missions to Mars. He'd been head of research at Schering Pharmaceuticals UK, a visiting professor at Sussex University, then a senior professor at the University of Zambia, as well as advising the World Health Organization's hormone research committee. Then there was his impressive list of publications.

If Deakin could attract high-flyers like Professor Michael Briggs, Jevons must have reasoned, whatever his reasons for being there might be, then the university could grow into the scientific centre of excellence he dreamed of. He seems to have thought that he had a lot in common with my dad, so he quickly became a close friend and ally. It was probably the unaccustomed glamour around this scientific celebrity that prevented Professor Jevons from being able to see the danger until it was too late.

Within a couple of years, Deakin had a disproportionately large and highly resourced biochemical research operation, in what was otherwise a small, non-specialist university. As his department steadily grew, the dean of sciences became increasingly powerful, controlling funding streams from several international pharmaceutical manufacturers. He gave personal assurances to the companies involved that the Deakin hormone laboratory could do all the specialist work they wanted, though the fees it would charge would be correspondingly high. His sphere of influence steadily increased, both inside and outside the university, as more and more money flowed in for research, particularly research about human and synthetic hormones.

In fact, the Deakin hormone laboratory only really existed in my dad's mind. It was just a name for the commercial activity he attracted into the faculty, but the executives who commissioned and paid for it had no reason to question that it existed.

After a while, the chair of the university ethics committee, Dr Jim Rossiter, heard rumours that were circulating among students and staff. Professor Briggs was making up research results without doing any experiments and diverting funds into his own bank account. A lot of what he was writing was being published in journals and books, so fake material was poisoning the ground for real researchers working on important hormone studies. Other invented data was sold directly to pharmaceutical companies, with a percentage of the profits being quietly skimmed off. Those pharmaceutical companies interpreted my dad's research as reassurance that their new products were safe and used it to support licensing applications and in advertising campaigns. It was a situation that was putting at risk the health and safety of potentially millions of women who were using the contraceptive pill, in many countries around the world.

My dad brushed off the concerns of senior members of the faculty, attributing their worries to inexperience. As the crisis escalated and pressure on him increased, my dad's affable façade started to crack. Until that point, he'd been a professor whose patent contradictions made him seem all the more appealing. He was erudite and scholarly, but he'd never lost his original accent and still spoke in the warm tones of a Manchester working man. Despite his intellectual achievements and his high status, he had the common touch, so he seemed genuine and natural. But according to an account published later by Jim Rossiter, this was not what he was like at their meetings, behind closed doors. He was aggressive, thin-skinned and serpentine, and prone to bouts of uncontrollable rage. Reports that my dad was not what he seemed only created further confusion: who or what was the real Professor Michael

Briggs, and what had he done? Jim Rossiter became increasingly marginalised as the investigation of my dad's alleged misconduct forced the campus community to take sides. Meanwhile, my dad slid into any perceived cracks in the social fabric of the university, opening them up further by charming a few of its more influential characters into his close confidence.

Two formal investigations collapsed in the face of convoluted legal strategies and pre-emptive strikes. But during the third committee of inquiry, when his critics were almost exhausted, my dad seems to have realised that he was too exposed to defend his position any longer. Very soon, he wasn't there to be investigated. And because he'd resigned without notice, the whole matter ended abruptly without any outcome at all.

Towards the end of the Australian winter of 1985, my dad flew via London to the dog days of August in a long, hot Spanish summer. He bought a fully furnished show house called Villa Valencia, in a half-built hillside development in Andalucia, overlooking Puerto Banus. He moved in with just a couple of suitcases.

4

A year later, the *Sunday Times* ran its exclusive 'The Bogus Work of Professor Briggs'. It took up several pages of the 'News in Focus' section and the story carried on in further articles in the *Times* and other papers in the UK and worldwide. It was the culmination of many months of research by investigative journalist Brian Deer, who had got wind of what might otherwise have seemed to be a purely internal problem for the ethics committee of a small university on the other side of the world. It was the first of several investigations by Brian Deer with scientific themes, which would go on to include the Andrew Wakefield MMR vaccine controversy, and the allegations of plagiarism that ended the media career of Dr Raj Persaud. My dad's international reputation and his advisory role with the World Health Organization, as well as the potential scale of a fraud involving international drug companies, probably made a local scandal into a major story. There was a reported 'leak' from Deakin University, which led to an initial flurry of interest in the Australian press. It was blamed for a while on Dr Jim Rossiter, but he said in turn that his office on campus had been broken into and documents relating to the investigation of my dad's conduct had been stolen.

The central allegation in the *Sunday Times* exposé was that my dad dishonestly claimed to have carried out the largest ever survey of long-term risks from the contraceptive pill. In fact, he'd taken the conclusions of very small studies by other people, then pretended he had obtained the same results from hundreds of women taking part in his studies. The companies that made the pills involved, Schering AG and Wyeth, had paid for the work through grants and were reliant on the data generated for licensing and marketing. Pharmaceutical companies had even funded large international symposiums where my dad could present his results from the podium with plenty of promotional fanfare, as well as publishing glossy textbooks for delegates. Government regulators in the UK had been persuaded to pass new pills which had supposedly been part of the study: the twenty-one-day dosage pill Logynon and the combined triphasic Trinordial. Similarly, the formulations Tri-Levlen and Triphasil were allowed to go on the market in the USA in part because of my dad's positive results.

It followed from the scale of the alleged scientific pretence that there must also have been financial fraud going on: it was unlikely that my dad was pretending to do research that was never done just to enrich Deakin University, so he must have been lining his own pockets. There were other, more peripheral, claims, and these painted a picture of wholesale wrongdoing and lack of integrity. For example, Brian Deer believed that my dad had lied about doing research using beagles. This could not be true, Deer reasoned, as there were no live dogs in the science department at Deakin University.

When Brian Deer had all the information he needed from sources in Australia and the USA, he went to find my dad in Spain, in the summer of 1986. There was a four-hour interview at Villa Valencia, during which Deer thought my dad had made some damning admissions. The article alleges that my dad admitted he hadn't organised studies himself but pretended that he had. He couldn't name the source of these results, or of other biochemical material he'd relied on. It's a basic problem for a scientist, not being able to show your working.

Dr Ursula Lachnit-Fixson, the head of Schering's medical research who was personally credited with the invention of the triphasic pill, didn't seem to have lost her faith in my dad as an authority in the field. She told Brian Deer that her company had: 'no reason whatsoever to doubt that his work has been done correctly'.

Brian Deer's meticulous pursuit of the story resulted in a very convincing case. Nonetheless, I think the beagle research accusation might not have been as well-founded as it had seemed at the time.

I'm not sure if Brian Deer knew about my dad's published work with Dr L N Owen, an animal pathologist at the University of Cambridge's Department of Veterinary Clinical Medicine. In their joint paper, 'Contraceptive Steroid Toxicology in the Beagle Dog and its relevance to human carcinogenicity' published in 1976, they concluded that beagles were not a good match for humans when testing the risk of breast cancer from hormonal medications, even though government regulators at the time required beagle studies to be done. Whatever was wrong with my dad and his research, the same can't be said of Dr Owen.

Dr Owen sourced the canine research samples used for the paper in 1976. One of the authors was in Geelong while the other was in Cambridge, doing different things, and that research did not require there to be a kennel full of dogs at Deakin's science department. The beagle research which added fuel to an already large fire in the 1980s was a later paper, 'Progestogens and mammary tumours in the beagle bitch', written by my dad in 1979. To a lay person, the articles seem very similar and I wonder if what my dad was guilty of was revisiting the earlier article to make the same point again. But in the grand scheme of things, it really doesn't matter. A long indictment might contain a few accusations that aren't proven, although the domino effect of guilt will lead in the end to the same verdict. It is a strange anomaly of my dad's story that this Owen and Briggs paper has remained in the scientific literature, as part of the specialist research output of Dr Owen. It's quite possible my dad believed he was a reputable 'man of science' like Owen, and enjoyed what he thought of as a collaboration of equals. But, left to his own devices, he couldn't sustain this version of himself for very long. And now, my dad's private science fiction was about to be exposed as a delusion.

After 28 September 1986, all my dad's own work was called into question because some of it was deliberately and provably flawed. The real-world consequence of what the *Sunday Times* had exposed was that millions of women taking contraceptive pills may not be safe, due to what my dad had done. In the aftermath of 'The Bogus Work of Professor Briggs', my dad faced the wiping-out of his carefully crafted identity as a trusted scientist.

5

After he left in 1970, there had been several long gaps when I'd chosen not to see my dad at all, though we exchanged short letters every so often. But when he moved back to Europe for the first time since I was nine years old, it seemed like the time had come to try to start again.

I was by then nearly twenty-three, an adult of sorts. I'd gone back to studying after a few years in temporary jobs, in fast-food restaurants and nightclubs. My A levels hadn't gone well, even though my chosen subjects had been what my dad had called 'an uncoordinated mishmash of soft options'. When I'd told him what I was planning to study this time, a mixed qualification called 'public administration', he said: 'Isn't that something people just do by accident?'

We met for lunch in London, near my birthday, in 1985. Then, the following summer, shortly before the publication of the *Sunday Times* exposé, I went to Andalucia to visit him in his new house.

Villa Valencia had been the first house to be built in what would become a large, gated development. It was at the end of an ancient donkey track, overlooking a steep, rubble-strewn slope leading down to a distant sprawl of white houses and the sea. I got out of the cab when the driver made it clear he would go no further, then I dragged my case for a further half-mile in the heat of the day. I let myself into a courtyard through a side gate. When I realised my dad wasn't there, I went into the grounds looking for a swimming pool.

I was drying myself with a towel from the pool house when my dad appeared, together with an old man I didn't know. When my dad introduced us, the man stared at me for a while and then said: 'I thought you said she was fat.'

By the time I got up the following morning, the man had gone. My dad was at the kitchen table, pouring coffee from a jug. His cup trembled against the saucer before he lifted it to his mouth. Then he said to the room, but not to me: 'He's a friend of a friend. He's been staying for a few days, but I don't really know him. I think he's got mild dementia, although from what I can gather, you could say, "He hath ever but slenderly known himself".'

'I'm sorry to hear that,' I said.

My dad reappeared a couple of hours after breakfast, smartened up, and suggested we go and sit on the north-facing terrace, behind the house, where we could stay out of the worst of the sun.

As we crossed the garden, he called out a few words in Spanish towards the man who had come to tend to the pool, who nodded back and smiled. The man was reattaching the pool filter to its corrugated tube, then he bent down and released it gently into the water, allowing it to wriggle away.

'There was a dog in the grounds when we arrived,' my dad said. 'A hunter's dog, I'd have thought, turned out into the wild. I called him Pedro. Andreas found him dead a few days ago, in the swimming pool. It took both of us to pull him out.'

'That's awful,' I said. 'Had he drowned?'

'Poisoned. The developers don't like strays.'

A large jug of rose-coloured liquid was set out on a table in the shade, with a couple of tumblers and a bowl of olives and almonds. He offered to pour me a glass.

'That's OK,' I said. 'You drink, I'll just cheers. I'll get myself a Coke when I go back inside.'

After a while, I asked him the question which had been in my mind since before I'd arrived. Why had he left his job and turned his back on Australia?

'Oh, I had no choice, I had to get out,' he said. 'The faculty, the staff, the Senate. All of them. Never hung poison on fouler toads than that lot, I can tell you.'

'But why did you come here?' I said. 'Spain's for holidays. Why not go back to England?'

He laughed. 'Oh, the weather!' he said. 'The weather, the rain. The constant, pouring rain.'

On the southern slope of the neighbouring hill, the next phase of construction was shimmering in a heat haze, bleached colourless by the intensity of the sun. The barren land around it was black from late-summer wildfires, dotted here and there with the burnt-out skeletons of wild yuccas.

'I can live anywhere I want. I've lived all over the world, as you know. I've had some adventures. My life's been like a film, some of it.'

'What in particular, has been like a film?' I asked.

'Ah, well,' he said. 'I could tell you, but then I'd have to kill you.' Then he laughed and looked away.

The scent of citrus oil mixed with tar drifted around on the hot dry air; fine ash from the wasted ground had started sticking to my reddened skin as soon as we'd gone outside. We listened in silence to the quiet sucking of the pool filter a short distance away, to the background rattle of crickets and to the distant grind of cement mixers.

'But, about Australia. And what happened. I'd been eating too much. And got a bit . . .' He patted his stomach, above the buckle of the belt on his shorts.

It wasn't obvious what he was trying to say, but he seemed to be trying to answer my original question.

'. . . on a lecture tour, in the United States. So, I went in early the following day, the day after I got back, and I parked off campus. To get a bit of exercise. There's a path just inside the boundary, though in places it's very overgrown. It's still bushland all around, everywhere beyond the fence.'

He seemed to lose the thread of what he was saying. He looked out across Villa Valencia's cultivated lawns, surrounded on three sides by a parched, blackish-brown desert, falling away at the back into a deep ravine. An army of sprinklers defended the hard green grass against the burning sun. But beyond the serpentine arcs of spray, on the other side of the chain-link fence behind the house, was a wilderness of thick, dry scrub.

'It was on the periphery road, close to the science block. I heard it first, before I saw it. There was a sound in the long grass, a rustling, on the other side of the fence.'

'What was it?' I said.

'Maybe a tiger snake or possibly a keelback, I couldn't tell. Once it was through the fence and in the open, I could see it was over three feet long. It coiled itself around so it could push itself forward, then it was right in my path. Then it rose up.'

He stiffened his forearm and pinched the tips of his fingers together into a cobra's head.

'It was stretching and swaying. Planning its next move, you might say, watching me. And then, suddenly, it struck.' He jabbed the puppet sharply towards my face, making me flinch.

He laughed again, letting his arm fall loosely to his side.

'There was a toad, a large cane toad. They're highly toxic, like snakes. The toad was behind me, in the rocks. The snake missed my ankle by a few inches and it went for the toad instead. It grabbed the toad by the head and pulled it out of its hiding place, holding it down. The toad screamed. A high-pitched scream, like a child. It fought back for a minute, then it was still. The snake was already eating it, long before it stopped moving. So, while it was swallowing, I knew I had to go.'

He gulped down his drink in a mouthful.

'After that, I never went back.'

'You mean, you never went back to the path by the fence?'

'No,' he said, 'I never went back to my office. Or to the university, in fact. There was no need to, anyway. So—'

'I don't understand. You just left . . . everything?'

He emptied the jug into his glass and set it aside.

'I did. There was just too much poison,' he said.

He lay back in his chair and closed his eyes.

'As Paracelsus said: it's not poison that kills you. It's the dose.'

❖ ❖ ❖

I watched a film on my own in the main house that evening. I think it was *Suddenly, Last Summer*. Then I walked back in the dark to the guest house by the pool, under the orange trees.

After that, the pattern of this life in Spain repeated daily. Nothing much happened. I lay by the pool and got a tan. One day, I heard a car outside and some people went into the house and were with my dad for several hours. Whether that was Brian Deer from the *Sunday Times*, I don't know. I wasn't told and had no reason to ask, at the time.

While he was drinking, my dad talked and I listened. A lot of it I'd heard before, all the weird science stories he used to like. Some of it was rambling, incongruous and bizarre. He said he'd had lots of affairs, one of them with a woman he named, who had become quite famous. Then there was his secret work for the British government, smuggling microfilm and a screw-together assassin's weapon across the Berlin Wall. The story about the affair with a minor celebrity sounded like it could be true. But I thought he'd probably seen the other thing in a James Bond film.

At the end of my visit, my dad stood with me at the roadside where the tarmac ended and the dust and stones began, until a taxi came to take me to the airport. I hugged him quickly before I climbed into the back seat, and instead of saying goodbye he said: 'I'd just wanted to tell him you were like me, that's all. But he took it the wrong way. Or maybe it didn't come out right.'

6

After I flew home from Spain, I heard nothing more from my dad for a while, which was not unusual. I found myself a job as an outdoor clerk in a solicitor's office, sitting in court taking notes, and making sure clients in the cells had clean shirts and cigarettes. Then, two months later, my dad suddenly reappeared.

He sent me a message, telling me to meet him at a restaurant in Brighton, not far from where I was working. It had once been a very popular place, and still had the baronial hall appearance and silver-service gentility that was fashionable when he'd taken me there once before, in the early 1970s. I waited for a while in the dark hallway until I was ushered through a heavy velvet curtain, although the dining room on the other side turned out to be almost empty, despite the time of day. A little weak sun fell through thickly leaded windows onto waiting white tablecloths, and flickering electric bulbs in cast-iron sconces on the walls were no more illuminating than real candles. In the half-light, I could just make out my dad, at a corner table. He was in character again, sitting alone, filling a wide carver chair to its sides.

I can't remember a time when my dad didn't look incongruous to me. His paradoxical absence and intimacy made him familiar and strange at the same time, like someone conjured into life from history or fiction. This time, he looked rather like a Tudor king waiting for his portrait to be painted. I sat down and asked him what he was doing here. He began stroking his face and neck with a large handkerchief and said after a long pause that there had been a 'misunderstanding'.

My dad owned several complete wardrobes of clothes, tailored to fit his fluctuating size, and that day he was wearing what must have been one of his largest pale blue seersucker suits. His characteristic tropical-executive style of dress tended to give him away as somebody from somewhere else, a place where the sun is always fiercely hot and bright, and suggested a protected life in perpetual transit between airport lounges, conference centres and air-conditioned hotels. His shoes were highly polished, almost certainly by somebody else. His ankles puffed out inside brightly coloured socks.

He put his handkerchief away in his trouser pocket and looked around as if he thought we might be overheard.

'It's just a misunderstanding but unfortunately it's all gone too far, so I've had no choice but to get the lawyers involved.'

He ordered for both of us without looking at the menu, while I asked him what kind of misunderstanding it was.

I'd wondered from time to time about the snake and the toad and what they might have meant, but this didn't seem to be the moment to bring it up. Had it been a metaphor? Was it a nightmare? Who might the snake be and who the toad? If they'd been real, had the snake been fatally poisoned when it swallowed the toad or had its toxic potential somehow increased?

'Oh, there's really nothing to it,' he said. 'It's just a pack of lies. But it will be sorted out by tomorrow, I should think.'

'Well, that's good,' I said.

'Academic life is full of professional jealousies,' he went on. 'Who should have had this, who was passed over for that, who's had more publications and preferments, who's giving a symposium. It's what keeps them all going, grinding away, looking over each other's shoulders. Then they bring it all to my door, to sort it all out for them. But it's all toxic.'

Covered plates arrived and the cloches were removed.

'So,' he said.

He ran a blunt knife down the seam of a dover sole and pulled apart the flesh into equal halves.

'What have you been up to?'

I'd been studying, of course. Then working. I could have told him I'd had my results since I last saw him, but only if I'd been prepared to explain it all again.

'Oh, nothing,' I said.

'Nothing?'

His fork moved rapidly from plate to mouth, and he chewed occasionally, not looking up.

'Yes,' I said. 'Nothing.'

'What you get for nothing,' he said, 'is nothing. You can see that, can't you?'

He wiped up pools of burnt butter with torn pieces of bread roll, working his way round methodically until there was none left.

'I'm not like you,' I said, after a while. 'I just look like you.'

He smiled, and I smiled as well.

'You see?' he said. 'That's exactly the point I'd been trying to make!'

Then he laughed, and sighed, calling me by my first name, shortened; a fatherly diminutive.

'I don't know,' he said. 'Though, in fact, I've taken a leaf out of your book myself.'

A waiter refilled his glass.

'I'd decided to retire anyway, even before all of this. Not stop completely. Just do what I want to. Write. Keep an Emeritus somewhere, probably. But I've no desire to lead anymore.'

I ate my fish as he drank and talked, although I wasn't very hungry.

'I will never understand the two of you,' he said. 'You and your brother. Both of you. Why neither of you has ever had my get up and go.'

Soon he changed the subject to more appealing topics. Like the microbiology of Jupiter, Creutzfeldt-Jakob disease in families who eat their ancestors, and his favourite undetectable deadly poisons.

Afterwards, I went to the platform with him and helped him onto the train.

'When's your meeting?' I said.

'Oh, not until five,' he replied. 'At Brick Court barrister's chambers.'

I waited so I could watch the train leave. As the whistle blew, he leaned down from the open window so I could put my face against his. Then I walked back to work, adding that moment to my small archive. Sample date: today, Friday. Sample type: warm skin, claret, cologne.

That became the final specimen in that collection.

Sometimes, in quiet moments, and over many years, I've gone back over that hour or so, to see if there was anything else that I should have noticed. I've wondered about what happened to him next, after the train pulled away. And whether there was something, anything, that might have explained what was really going on. And why I would never see him again.

7

Friday, 26 September 1986

After saying goodbye at the station, Michael edged along the swaying corridor until he found an empty compartment. Seeing his daughter, even for a short time, was unsettling. He was never sure if she set out to provoke him, or if she was able to catch him off-guard through some strange intuition. Maybe she's more like her mother than she looks, he thought. He closed the sliding door from the corridor and settled down beside the window with his back to the engine, then he opened the folder of court papers, with every intention of reading them.

But he didn't. He'd started playing around with this meeting in his mind as soon as he'd been told about it, rehearsing it this way and that way. He'd enjoyed polishing his performance, refining it by repetition, and the fantasy lured him irresistibly back once more.

'You know I'm a man with an unimpeachable reputation,' he'd decided to say, probably looking up from the grand conference table, making eye contact with his solicitor and then with his Queen's Counsel. 'And that I'm an internationally recognised expert in my field. With the highest academic qualifications from the great universities, and many hundreds of publications to my name.'

Then he thought he'd pause, to underline the point, and to demonstrate his sincerity and the depth of his concern.

'And therefore,' he'd continue, perhaps looking down again, 'fighting back isn't a choice. I have to stop the poison from spreading; I have to see off the green-eyed monsters. And surely, if I really was a fraud, like they say' – here he would smile at such a patently ridiculous suggestion – 'then, why has there never been any evidence of it before?'

He would tell the judge that he was motivated only by a life-long pursuit of the truth. Monetary damages were, for him, a very minor concern: 'I'm here to clear my name, that's all. There will need to be retractions and apologies, of course. From all of them, all the journals, all the papers, all my accusers.

'Hand on heart,' he would say, with his hand resting on his heart, 'my innocence is a simple, provable fact. So, let's get all this over and done with, once and for all.'

Suing a national newspaper would be a high-stakes gamble – his solicitor had already said so. Asking a judge to gag a free press was a very risky strategy indeed, in every possible way. But as the train sped through the Sussex countryside, Michael dismissed this concern with a wave of his hand.

'I'm not worried at all because I'm telling the truth. Tell the truth and shame the devil, as my mother would say.'

Then they'll laugh and they'll shake hands. The conference will be over. They'll set off for the Royal Courts of Justice for a midnight injunction. He'll silence them all: Jim Rossiter, Brian Deer. Rupert Murdoch. All of them.

The law would be his friend again, Michael thought to himself. As it had been at Deakin, at least to start with. The law would be there again to protect his reputation, and his secrets.

There was no reason he could think of why it wouldn't.

8

In late September of 1986, two days after I'd left my dad at the station, I went out to buy a newspaper. I took a *Sunday Times* off the top of the pile, which was next to a similar stack of copies of the *News of the World*. The *News of the World* had a typical red-top headline, which I was about to find out was a plug for the main story in its stablemate at News International, the *Sunday Times*: 'Bogus Boffin Is Unmasked'.

I think both papers had the same small picture on the front cover, though it was a long time ago. It fitted into a single column of print and was of a man who looked exactly like my dad. It was a teaser for what was inside. On the cover of the next section, my dad's life-size, black and white face bore the stamp of the accusation, in capital letters.

I don't remember any kind of emotion, though my heart was racing as I read it. I'd learned in childhood to step back from strong feelings around this unpredictable parent, to move away and watch. So that probably wasn't surprising.

'That's intriguing,' my brother said later.

'I assume he's back in Spain,' I said. 'But I've no idea. I'd ring him up if he had a phone. But he hasn't. The wires haven't stretched as far as Villa Valencia. It's in the middle of a building site, halfway up a mountain.'

'What did he say when you saw him on Friday?'

'Well, hardly anything, really. Only that there'd been a "misunderstanding", as he called it.'

'I'm not sure that really covers it,' my brother said.

'And he'd come over here to try and sort it out.'

'Not entirely successfully, as it turns out. I wonder what he'll do now?'

'He'll sue, I should think, if he hasn't already. He'll have to, now. I know he was seeing some lawyers after he saw me, but I assumed it was just about some row he left behind in Australia. It's obviously gone in the papers anyway. He hasn't got a choice, surely? His whole reputation will be ruined. Maybe it already is.'

'From the article, I'd say he's bang to rights. He seems to have admitted most of it.'

'He was drinking a lot when I saw him in Spain in July. And quite a bit at lunch the other day as well. I think he's seen it coming for a while.'

'The papers are saying he's got plenty of money, mainly in backhanders. Mum always thought he had more than he let on, squirrelled away in Switzerland or something. So maybe he doesn't need to work.'

'The final straw for him seems to have been something to do with a snake. On the way to his office. And a poisonous toad.'

'Are you joking?' my brother snorted.

'No, honestly. He said a big snake and a cane toad stopped him from going back to his office. He told me about it when I was in Spain.'

'I must try that myself, next time I don't want to go some-where. He's really scared of snakes, though. Which is a bit strange for a toxicologist, though maybe you can know too much about some things. He won't go near them, even in the zoo.'

'He must be really stressed, that's all. Maybe he's started seeing things.'

'Maybe he's been licking toads,' my brother said.

'Or alternatively, he's gone totally nuts.'

❖ ❖ ❖

Reassuring announcements about contraceptive safety popped up on the television and in the press over the next few weeks. A parliamentary committee was set up to look into it. The World Health Organization advised all the women affected to carry on following their doctor's advice. I watched the news along with everyone else; I was an interested user of the triphasic pill myself, as well as the daughter of what might soon be a wanted man. I wondered if my dad was already on the run, as I'd heard nothing more from him.

On the popular science show *Tomorrow's World*, there was the same close-up of my dad's face, but this time blown-up to enormous size and hanging from the studio ceiling. I looked at the face and I thought: you don't know him. None of you know him. There, there's the mole on his cheek he catches sometimes when he's shaving, then he'll patch the cut with a torn scrap of tissue paper. Here, here's the deep cleft in his chin. If this picture wasn't in black and white, you could see that his eyes are intense, pale blue. That's my dad. He's *my* dad. And he's in an awful lot of trouble.

9

Whenever I catch a train from the station that's closest to where I still live, I pass the spot where I last saw my dad, not far off forty years ago. Other passengers walk through the place without being aware of its significance, because that's all it is: a place on a station platform.

I hardly ever stand in it and say: *Are you there?*

So. Are you?

Am I what?

Are you there?

In a way, I am. But only like Wells's time machine.

How would that be?

If you remember, when the Morlocks steal the time machine, they drag it away into the pyramid.

I do remember that, in the film. I watched it with you.

My point is that when the traveller arrives home to his own time, the time machine is in his front garden, rather than his study. The garden and the study are in the same spaces and in the same relationship to each other as the place where the time machine had been, and the pyramid. But the house and garden are there in 1900, not 800,000 years later. Do you see?

I think so. You are still there. But just not now. It's the right place, but not the right time.

When I catch the train to London, from the carriage window I can see what he would have seen from the train that day. One of the stations on the line would have triggered a memory. It's very near to where we used to live, in the 1960s. Following the brook over the field then through the trees will take you to the last house where we lived together as a family. The station was quiet then. Trains still sometimes go through it without stopping.

My parents moved to this place when I was about three years old, then, when they separated, my mother took my brother and me to live by the coast, a few miles away. She bought a house and later a shop in the small village where I now live. I have an invisible tie to that place too; but not, I don't think, to her.

A short distance from my mother's house, and from mine, there's a steep slope down to a grey shingle beach. The beach is divided into sections by stone groynes and separated from the rest of the world by tall white cliffs. A slippery chalk reef is exposed at low tide, where small crabs, sand fleas and anemones inhabit temporary rockpools. A higher tide can be benign, bright blue-green and still. Or it can be dark and destructive, loud and wild. Or it can dissemble, pretending to be what it is not, to catch you out if you get too close.

My mother went down to this beach every evening. She'd pick up stones with naturally occurring holes through them, called hag stones, and keep them in her pockets. People who earned their living from the sea often did the same, before the rising tide of scientific certainty washed away their magic.

Through the hole in a hag stone, you can see the world as it should be, stripped of cunning deceptions, without artifice. The hole is also an irresistible lure, an impassable witch-trap. Witches of every kind can't stop themselves from diving in and getting themselves stuck.

10

In July 2020, the Cumberlege report had revived some fragmented memories. I wanted to find out everything I could about my dad's newly discovered connection with this newly discovered controversy over the drug Primodos. I picked up another newspaper the following day, in the same newsagent's where I'd bought the *Sunday Times* in late September of 1986. Like the traveller inside the pyramid, I was in the same space in another time. I wanted to see his name again, or even another photograph.

When something like this had happened before, most of my life was still in front of me. My dad had been alive, though on borrowed time. As I queued up outside the shop in a cloth mask, I thought about how much he would have enjoyed the novelty of a worldwide pandemic.

What do you think about Covid, Dad?

Not a wholly negative development, I don't think.

Why so?

Well, I'd say a novel disease is just the opportunity we need to demonstrate our immunological superiority over Martians. If it wasn't for good old earthly pathogens, Woking would still be overrun with alien tripods.

The pandemic had felt like *The War of the Worlds* at times. The virus restrictions still prevented people from gathering inside, so both the village cafes were closed. I took my paper down to the beach instead, where the salt air felt fresh and un-infectious, and people had started to behave more normally again. On the way, I paused for a moment outside my mother's house, long since sold to new owners. It's tall, narrow and very old, made from eighteenth-century rubble, grey flints and tarred wood, and with a simple, childish shape, like a toy building on a model railway.

Daisy-like pink and white fleabane had seeded itself into the walls and was beginning to flower between the flints, pushing out broken pieces of dry mortar. My mother always said fleabane kept evil spirits at bay.

I'd been sitting on the shingle for some time, immersed in scanning and turning the pages, when I heard a voice say: 'Can you take my picture for me?'

I looked up and saw a young woman standing nearby, holding up her phone in front of her unmasked face. It used to be common to be asked by strangers to take photos, but not so much these days. She looked no more than twenty-five and unlikely to need any help from me to take a picture, but she was on her own and I think she was bored. A kind of nervous energy had been released into public spaces by the relaxation of the coronavirus lockdown. We were all a bit lonelier than we were before and it was a relief to be able to interact again, but chatting with strangers might be unwelcome and transgressive, possibly even illegal.

'Yes, of course,' I said. An unexpected gust of wind ruffled the pages of my newspaper, so I picked up a stone to weight them down. I didn't notice the hole until it was already in my hand.

'I've taken a selfie, but I can't get the sea and the cliffs.'

'It's no trouble,' I said, taking the phone from her for a moment then passing it back.

'Are you from round here?' she asked.

'Yes, my late mother lived here for years. I used to play on this beach sometimes when I was a kid.'

She was studying the picture I'd just taken, on the screen of her phone.

'I'm not,' she said. 'But I think it's allowed, for exercise or something. This is such a pretty beach. You've probably got lots of photos of you here, from when you were younger?'

I could see she was imagining mezzotints of the mid-century olden days, of which I was obviously a living relic.

It would have to have been after 1970, of course. And after 1970, the photos fizzled out. I could only think of two, in a paper bag stuffed with loose snaps. In each of them, my mother is in the foreground with my brother and me only just visible behind her, out of focus. They were taken by a man who had been interested in her, but after a few days out I don't think it went any further. He had a fancy 35mm camera, and I suspect his chosen focal distance reflected deeper misgivings about starting a relationship with a woman with children.

'Not many,' I said. 'It wasn't that kind of family.'

'What was your mum like?' she asked.

I picked up the hag stone and looked back at her through the hole.

'Oh, you know,' I said. 'A bit mad.'

❖ ❖ ❖

My mother was already grieving the unexpected loss of her marriage when she discovered she'd been turned against her will into a single parent, like a curse in a fairy story. Her understanding of everyday life had always admitted the possibility of being bewitched, so when, as she saw it, a powerful malignancy locked the three of us in a high tower with no door, I think she was very disappointed but not particularly surprised. Enchanted brambles sprang up rapidly all around us, obscuring the windows and blocking her only means of escape, but my mother sustained herself with a magical inner life, full of hidden patterns and secrets.

Like William Blake on Peckham Rye, my mother was able to see angels in the ordinary world. They were visually indistinct and fluid, but they were nonetheless there, and sometimes they would comment on her circumstances, without going so far as to offer any help or advice. She saw a lot of angels during a period of unexplained illness which began suddenly when I was a baby. It was severe hypercalcaemia – an abnormally high concentration of calcium in the blood – which came close to killing her. But once she'd recovered sufficiently to be no longer in danger, she discovered an idiosyncratic spirituality in her near-death experiences that was in many ways the same as a formal religion.

My brother was immune to supernatural thinking and I looked to him as a pillar of sanity. Sometimes we talked about the likelihood that our mother was mad, though in all these discussions I kept quiet about having committed most of what she told me to memory. It seemed to me remotely possible there was some method in it. Maybe there were things I needed to know buried somewhere in there, if only I could find them.

My mother believed she had special powers, although she didn't think of her talents as occult, but rather more like being naturally musical or good at sums. She had vivid childhood memories in which she rose up from the furniture then fluttered, moth-like, against the ceiling, but whenever I tried this myself I had very little success. Maybe I was too heavy or lacked the necessary strength of faith. My mother used bibliomancy to help her to make important decisions, and while we had several different religious texts as well as a copy of the I-Ching in the house, she was just as likely to get prophetic insights by going to the bookshelf and randomly opening *Zen and the Art of Motorcycle Maintenance*, *The Rubaiyat of Omar Khayyam*, *A Christmas Carol* or the Yellow Pages.

My mother's inner certainty made her convincing to others who otherwise ought to have known better, not just me. Because she never doubted, for example, that she could cure warts by buying them with copper coins, there were people who swore this had worked when all other treatments had failed. She had been unable to cure herself of hypercalcaemia, but luckily her childhood invisible friend returned in the mid-1960s in the form of a Jordanian doctor in the ward called Yahia Dajani, who was instrumental in her miraculous recovery. The invisible friend had been called Yehyeh; he'd disappeared unexpectedly in 1940, but in his time, he'd had his own chair and a place was set for him at every meal. Yehyeh's connection with Dr Dajani was not entirely rejected by the doctor, whose rational sense was temporarily overborne by my mother's unusual charm. She believed Yehyeh disappeared so he could be born in human form as Yahia. His pre-existence with a similar name must have involved complicated theology or convoluted theoretical physics, but that didn't need to be explained to be understood.

My mother's system of belief was underpinned by predestination narratives and origin myths, with roots in our recent family history and infused with magical meanings. As I grew up,

I learned all about my parents' first meeting, the films they saw, the great ships on which they travelled, and what they did in Canada, America and New Zealand in their early married life. Starting from the outing to the pictures to see *The Incredible Shrinking Man*, I became the keeper of the only known record of their relationship. It was a jumbled testament, with a loose structure of real events tangled together with rambling allegory and exotic varieties of mysticism.

In spite of everything that happened, my mother never lost her unshakeable belief in my father's genius, which made his cruelty towards her that much harder to bear. Sometimes she would sing a jazz-age ballad about travelling west, 'Home in Pasadena', which conjured up the happy times they'd had together in Pasadena, California, in the early 1960s, as if the loving husband and the man who had left her were two completely different people.

I want to be a home-sweet-homer, there I'll settle down,
Beneath the palms in someone's arms, in Pasadena town.

When lack of money forced the sale of the last house where we'd lived as a family, my mother went out and trapped a large toad in a bucket on the wet ground by the brook, releasing her that night under the gate and into the yard of the empty cottage she wanted to buy. The toad looked after the property on my mother's behalf until contracts could be exchanged, while eating her fill of garden pests in the overgrown rockery. I don't know what became of the toad after we moved in: my brother and I didn't spend much time outside as there was little out there to do.

In a different time and place, my mother would have been a productive and successful artist, but she had to find practical work to keep the three of us once my dad was no longer there. She went back to cutting patterns and making clothes, and she was more skilful with line and colour than you would have guessed from what she was paid. In the rest of her waking hours, she drew figures in charcoal, then sculpted them in clay. She filled hundreds of notebooks with ink and wash sketches of ordinary life, viewed as if through a hag stone, stripped of artifice. Sometimes she painted huge canvases of things she alone could see. But there was never enough time for any of that.

I wanted to believe in a world that worked in the way my mother thought it did. But it seemed likely that my mother's eccentricity, her irrationality even, had driven my dad away and she was to blame for that. I rarely considered the alternative, that he was the more culpable, because he wasn't the one who was there. We were told he had been spirited away by a woman, who was herself a scientist. A little older, childless and, I imagined, intellectually his equal, but with the added gift of feminine tricks and deceptions. I had no doubt that she must be the source of the curse that had fallen on us and held us captive, never my dad. He was too brilliant to be troubled by trivial, worldly things.

From my small and sometimes precarious vantage point, I observed at a distance what I understood to be my dad's continuing rise to prominence, as if watching a distant comet. He seemed to me to be rare, enigmatic, powerful and very far away. I sometimes imagined him in places that I thought might suit him – a benign and silent ghost of himself, standing by a window looking out or sitting in the chair in my room, reading.

11

So, in the summer of 2020, I began the search for my elusive dad all over again. But rather than looking for him in shadowy corners or empty chairs, this time I could go online. I found my old box file of yellowing *Sunday Times* newspaper cuttings from 1986 and I laid them out on the table next to my laptop. I was curious to see if there was anything I'd missed the last time: an obvious clue I'd overlooked, when I'd been unaware how much there was that I didn't know.

I turned over the page and saw the black letters partly obscuring his face, after a gap of many years. He was looking out at me through a narrow slit in time, as if through prison bars. In this old newspaper, I could see how my dad was pinned down, close to the end. In the article, he's trapped forever on the threshold of an ancient disaster, doomed to repeat its perpetual loop of actions and gestures.

In 'The Bogus Work of Professor Briggs', Brian Deer describes pulling up outside my dad's house, as the police might do in a cop drama. Deer could see that my dad had anticipated and feared this turn of events. I'd forgotten that he'd been doorstepped in this way, like a criminal. But then I suppose there were plenty of people who'd say he was not much less than a criminal. Fraud is a crime, after all, though the larger and more impressive it is, the less likely the perpetrator is to see the inside of a jail cell. And my dad's turn of phrase was that of a cornered but unrepentant felon:

'If I tell you who organised the studies you will know who is involved,' he says. *'And I'm not prepared to drop people in it.'*

His original accent, never lost, could well have been a subliminal influence acting in his favour. As a highly respected expert who sounded like someone ordinary, he could give simple, honest-sounding answers to complicated questions. But now he was saying he wouldn't 'drop people in it', sounding like any other suspect might do in a Manchester custody suite.

Then, when my dad was on the point of breaking down in tears, he cried out: 'What am I supposed to do?' He'd finally been cornered, in a position he felt unable to explain, from which he would never be able to extricate himself. But, even then, he still didn't name names.

That summer in Andalucia, the same summer as this interview, I'd felt sorry for my dad for the first time in my life. He'd been weakened by something and at times he seemed out of his mind. My child-changed father had provoked protective instincts in me. But this interview, a four-hour grilling, was altogether more mysterious. Not for what my dad said but what he didn't say, despite the unbearable pressure he was under.

I allowed my eyes to flick backwards and forwards, reading a line or two of print then looking up again at the screen, at the long list of search titles and terms. I picked up and followed lead after lead, going down paths into dead ends. Then I followed a thin thread to an article in a far corner of the internet. It was 'Reflections of a Whistle-Blower' by Jim Rossiter, the head of the Deakin University ethics committee, and had been published in 1992, a few years after the cuttings on the table next to me.

Jim Rossiter felt he'd been obstructed at every turn when he tried to investigate my dad's forceful character and unorthodox behaviour. But he also said he'd been personally threatened and intimidated in hundreds of silent telephone calls and obscene letters threatening him with blackmail. In this strangely angled sidelight on the past, Rossiter described a remorseless bully who lacked any kind of moral restraint. Who was, according to him, my dad. This was not a perspective on my dad that I had ever imagined, which raised the possibility that there was a very different side to him that had always been hidden from view. Perhaps even connected with what he may have been concealing during the Brian Deer interview.

Jim Rossiter certainly believed my dad perpetrated a vicious campaign of harassment against him. It hadn't been proved at the time, there was no appetite to do so, and now there was no remaining evidence of it. But there was another serious allegation in Rossiter's paper which could still be verified and could only be either true or false.

Jim Rossiter was convinced that my dad had no right to be on the academic staff of a university, let alone to hold a professorial chair.

Rossiter believed that my dad had lied about his qualifications, and that he was a charlatan.

12

As a founding dean at Deakin University, my dad had been allowed to choose where his office would be, in the early days while the university was still under construction. He picked a position in a quiet corner of the campus close to the site perimeter, away from the bustle of students and the prying eyes of colleagues. Over the years, he'd decorated it with the proof of his achievements, so its walls were covered with copperplate certificates from grateful collaborators and its shelves were filled with his own publications. But at the peak of the research scandal in 1985, he left his office one day and he never went back, as if he had developed a sudden aversion to it. For several months after he left the university, my dad's office on campus remained as it had been when he'd locked the door for the last time.

Some letters from this episode in the life of the university, which became known as 'the Briggs affair', have been preserved in Deakin's archives, so a small amount of tangential evidence still exists about what happened next.

In January 1986, the door was opened with a skeleton key and what was left was packed up into crates, so the room could be used by the newly appointed replacement dean of sciences. The letters show that the university registrar wrote to my dad asking what should be done with all his belongings. Five months passed without any response, so the boxes were removed and put into storage. Another letter was sent in July 1986, by air mail certified delivery to my dad's home in Spain.

On 14 August 1986, the registrar decided to try one last time. He wrote again and eleven days later, my dad wrote back. He instructed the registrar that 'all the books should go to the library, the reprints of articles should go to whoever might want them, and the rest to be destroyed.'

The registrar must have gone to the repository, to do as he'd been asked. He would have approached this task methodically, I'm sure, stacking up reference books and articles, and throwing out photographs, letters and postcards, as well as an accretion of pharmaceutical merchandise – the branded paperweights, pens, notepads and executive toys that I'd seen on my dad's desk during a visit to Australia a few years before. Then he must have come across two objects that were not in the category to be preserved. He'd have wondered for a while what he should do with them. But he must have decided to set them aside.

'Surely, Professor Briggs must have forgotten they were there,' the registrar probably thought to himself.

On 24 November 1986, the registrar posted a parcel with a note inside, confirming that in every other respect he had complied with my dad's wishes. But among his belongings, he had found these two things and he felt in all conscience that he couldn't put them on the bonfire.

Inside the parcel was a Doctor of Philosophy thesis from 1959, *A Study of Biotin and its Analogues*, bound in blue cloth. And a slimmer volume of the same size, a Doctor of Science thesis, dated 1961 and bound in red.

My dad was probably still alive when the parcel was posted in Australia, but he was almost certainly dead by the time it was delivered to Villa Valencia, so he never saw what was inside or read the note. Whether he'd wanted the blue and red theses to be burned with everything else is very hard to say. But if he'd remembered they were still in his office at Deakin, it's very likely that he did. He alone knew that these documents were not what they pretended to be. And as the risk of exposure steadily increased, so did their potential to harm him.

I don't know exactly what happened to them next, after they arrived too late in Spain, but they continued to exist after their author did not.

13

I ring my brother again.

'It's your sister here.'

'I know,' he says. 'What can I do for you?'

'What do we know about Dad's qualifications?' I ask him. 'I mean, his paper qualifications, his degrees?'

'Well, as far as I'm aware, he took his first degree at Liverpool, in chemistry. That's when Mum and Dad met of course, sometime in the late fifties. And we know he then got a PhD in America, from Cornell in New York State. And, after that, a Doctor of Science from Wellington in New Zealand. Round about when I was born. 1961.'

'But how do we know that?' I say.

'I suppose because he told us he did, or Mum probably did. Or both. But mainly because I've got the last two, here in my office. There's a blue one and a red one. I'm looking at them now, they're next to my thesis as a matter of fact, on the same shelf. I'm not even sure how I got them.'

My brother has worked on his own for over twenty years, unable to tolerate the noise and unwelcome social interactions that were the byproducts of life in a university mathematics department. He nurtures a homemade system of odds-processing software which earns him a comfortable living, mainly from horse-racing, and sometimes he leaves the house to go to a betting shop, to see if he can improve on technology using more old-fashioned techniques. Every so often, he will have a steak breakfast at a windowless local casino and then play blackjack, but only if the cards are dealt in the traditional way, from a shoe with fewer than eight packs. He counts cards because he is unable not to, and to him it is as much a part of the game as judging how much he can win without attracting attention. I believe he counts everything and sometimes it makes him money. When people ask what my brother's job is, I usually say 'professional gambler', which conjures up an image wholly at odds with reality: it makes him sound slick and persuasive with an easy, superficial charm, like a flashily dressed con artist from a story by Damon Runyon or Graham Greene.

When I get to his house, my brother is dressed as usual in army surplus shorts held up with an elastic belt, blue Crocs and grey, shin-length socks. The visible hem of an ill-fitting patterned shirt separates his casual lower half from that part of him which is planning to attend an online meeting. He pauses only for long enough to open the front door and is already walking away down the hall as I come in, continuing our earlier conversation as he goes. I follow him to his study.

'Here they are,' he says. And we stand side by side, looking at them.

The two theses laid out on his desk are both standard hardback volumes, A4 in size but of differing thicknesses, bound in cloth. The thicker one is blue, the other a dark maroon-red, and each is stamped with Dad's name on the spine in gold letters as well as a date: 1959 and 1961 respectively. The blue one has a subject title, an award and a location on its cover, also in gold: *Studies of the Biochemistry of Biotin and its Analogues. Cornell*

University PH.D. A couple of Dad's earliest published books, the only ones we own, have been placed beside them: *A Handbook of Philosophy*, published in Canada when Dad was twenty-four, and *Current Aspects of Exobiology*, a collection of papers about possible life-forms elsewhere in the universe, published in 1966.

'So, what do you think he did this time around?' my brother says, picking up the blue book and opening it.

'I really don't know,' I say. 'He was responsible for Primodos being on the market, for a few years anyway. Primodos was given to women by GPs from their desk drawers, and some people think it caused a lot of pain and misery.'

'What was it doing in the GP's desk drawer?' he says.

'I'm not sure about that either. It's what a lot of the women say happened to them. But actually, I don't know. Maybe the point is that it wasn't properly regulated. Or there were a lot of free samples washing around. But you don't usually get medicines from a desk drawer, do you?'

I pick up the other volume, the red one.

'The thing is, we always knew there was something about our dad that wasn't quite right, didn't we? We just couldn't quite work out what it was.'

I open the book, and look at the first page: *Dr Briggs is married, with one son.*

14

I decided to see if I could find the reference copy of my dad's PhD in the only place it could be: Cornell University library. It was possible, even likely, that it would still be somewhere in the university's archives. Within a few minutes, I'd found something listed in the online catalogue by Michael H Briggs, with the same title as the blue thesis on my brother's desk, *Studies on the Biochemistry of Biotin and its Analogues*, and with the same date, September 1959. I emailed the librarian and asked them to send me some images of it. The fact that it was there was reassuring.

Whatever else my dad might have done, it would at least prove that Jim Rossiter was wrong.

❖ ❖ ❖

The following day, screen shots arrived from the Cornell librarian of the first few pages of the thesis I'd seen in the library catalogue, as well as a picture of the spine and front cover. As I worked out how to make the thumbnail images bigger, I wondered if this book had been untouched and unvisited on a shelf in Ithaca, New York, for all the intervening decades. The last person to have opened it before now could easily have been my dad, before he left it there for safe keeping sometime in the late summer of 1959. My mother, still only twenty-three years old, would have been packing their tin trunk somewhere, getting ready for the next part of their adventure together, 9,000 miles away in New Zealand.

The pictures were of a thesis very similar to the one that I'd taken from my brother's desk. It was almost the same in fact, but not quite.

On the title page of our copy, it says: *A thesis presented to the Graduate School of Cornell University for the degree of Doctor of Philosophy, September 1959.* But the library version, the true copy, is just a master's dissertation, written at the end of a course of lectures. It isn't a doctorate at all.

A single-page biography is also missing from the counterfeit thesis we've inherited, which sets out the true sequence of events. My dad describes in it how he'd gone to Cornell in the September of 1958 to study for a Master of Science degree. And how he'd supported himself and my mother by working for three terms as a teaching assistant.

My dad had been a student at Cornell for only one academic year. And the blue book in the parcel, somehow delivered to my brother from Australia via Spain, was a carefully constructed theatrical prop – or perhaps the small, believable detail that lends credibility to a much bigger confidence trick.

He'd removed the original hard covers, which seemed from the pictures to have been the same shade of blue, then he must have created a few new pages before putting the whole manuscript back together as something new. I zoomed in, to blow up a recurring idiosyncrasy in the type to full screen, trying to compare it with the corresponding pages in the fabricated version next to me. He seemed to have used the same typewriter. Probably his own portable.

He'd lied to everyone, from his colleagues and employers to his children. To the bookbinder who was his unknowing accessory.

'Oh, you know what scientists are like!' he'd have said. 'I never had the time or the money to get it made up properly.

But now. Now that I've got myself a shelf to put it on . . .' He'd have smiled, in a shy display of pride.

I'm not sure how I would have felt if I'd found this out when my dad was still alive. When everything I did was never good enough. When I didn't try hard enough. When I failed to show any promise. Proving, as we'd both agreed, that I wasn't destined go far.

But the fact is, I'm a great deal older now than he was then, when he devoted so much attention and care to the first big deception of his career. And the woman I've become isn't angry with him. I'm more intrigued.

15

'In retrospect, we should probably have been more suspicious a long time ago,' my brother says. 'It just wasn't plausible that he knew everything he said he did. I doubt there's been a "man who knew all science" since Copernicus. There's just too much of it these days.'

I meet up with my brother a week after the email from Cornell, walking our dogs. We always follow my brother's preferred route and go at the same time of day. We take the track across a field, through some woods, past an old sheep pond and loop back along the side of a golf course.

Dog walking provides an opportunity to talk outside the normal world as brother and sister, without any of the social barriers created by face-to-face conversation.

'Surely it was other people who should have been suspicious first,' I say. 'How could we possibly have known if he was making things up?'

'We were just children, that's true,' my brother says. 'And if several universities, Schering Pharmaceuticals and the World Health Organization just accepted it all at face value, then I suppose we were in good company. But now we know he never did any original research at Cornell, only a taught-course master's. And that, at some point, he decided to create his own PhD thesis, though we don't know when or why.'

We arrive at a fork in the path that he passes every day, where two crows are waiting for him. He takes a handful of dog biscuits from his pocket and the crows rise with them simultaneously into the air.

'Then, once there is *one* provable fake,' he continues, 'then you have to wonder about the other one. The Doctor of Science degree. Supposedly he got that in 1961, only two years later. A DSc is a super-doctorate, it's like a lifetime achievement award, not something you get at whatever age he was.'

'Twenty-six,' I say. 'He was twenty-six when he applied, in 1961, twenty-seven the following August. Dad was very plausible, though, wasn't he? He was a smooth talker. And it probably suited everyone to go along with what he said. I think that's a natural reaction.'

My brother picks up a stick and throws it out across the water, as the dogs head off together into the pond, with my older one lagging a little way behind.

'When we were kids, he always told incredible stories about science. And he talked about space like he'd just got back from Jupiter the day before.'

'There's nothing wrong with liking space,' my brother says. 'I got you out of bed to see the moon landing in sixty-nine. Space was very fashionable in those days.'

'I'm sure he had fantasies about being a famous scientist, back when he was young. Flash Gordon would have been on at the Saturday-morning pictures. *Journey into Space* was on the radio as well. But he was a working-class boy from a northern mill town. He was the first person in his family to go to university. He had no money, no connections of any kind. Maybe he faked the

PhD because didn't think he had the time to waste, doing it properly. Then he got ahead, so he carried on cutting corners, taking the odd liberty. And he got luckier, and he didn't get caught. Then maybe he just forgot. He forgot that he wasn't the highly decorated and esteemed scientist he'd convinced everybody else he was.'

'Would he ever have done any of that stuff, though?' my brother says. 'The NASA Mars probe, research director of an international drug company, whatever. If he hadn't been a fraud?'

'Well, no,' I say. 'That's presumably why he had to carry on with the lie. Otherwise, he would have had to get a normal job, like other people's dads. A lab technician, maybe. Or a schoolteacher, like he originally planned.'

We walk on in silence for a while.

'And what was the job in between, in Wiltshire?' I ask. 'When I was born. When we lived in Chippenham?'

'I can only remember there being a cow, and if you'd asked me what it was like I'd have said it had a hole in it. But that must be nonsense. Cows don't have holes in them, do they? I certainly can't tell you why he'd have had a single cow, with or without a hole in it.'

'What was it like, where we used to live?' I ask. 'I don't remember.'

'The two houses were very similar, the first one in Wiltshire and the second one in Sussex,' my brother says. 'And more like the house they'd just left in Pasadena than an English house would usually be. They were new, big, all on one level, detached, with gravel driveways and a big front lawn. Expensive, I'd imagine. But the second one was better, because it had a brook, in the dip between the end of the garden and the field behind. You remember that? It isn't very far from a little station, you can almost see the house from the Victoria train, not very far from the airport either, but still surrounded by fields. The brook was more of a muddy ditch, really. You didn't like it in the brook, but you'd sit on the bank and watch when I got in there. There were loads of frogs, toads, sticklebacks, that kind of thing. And spawn. I gave you a coffee jar full of spawn, with a loose lid. But you spilt it all down the underfloor heating vent. Do you remember?'

16

I turned the blue and red books over and over in my hands, opening and closing them, trying to put myself in the mind of the man who made them. I wondered if, by close reading, or even by using some of my mother's bibliomancy, they might provide the key that finally unlocked the secret code. Maybe if I understood why they existed I'd see my dad clearly at last, without artifice.

But it wasn't very likely to work that way, if that was even something I truly wanted. I was used to the façade and was becoming increasingly less sure that I'd like what was concealed behind it. The books were part of a disguise that after a while had started to slip, and that was when Jim Rossiter had seen something very ugly underneath.

The first, the blue fake, fitted so neatly with its red companion that it was very hard to believe the red one could possibly be real. The consequence of neither being real would of course be that Dr Michael Briggs had been plain Mr Briggs all along, rising to worldwide fame in the scientific community with no reason to be there at all. Then there was Primodos. Unlike all the academic papers and the theoretical trips to Mars, Primodos had always had the potential to hurt real people.

If I could find an evidence trail, I thought, then the timing of the fraud might reveal what the real point of it had been. Immediate fabrication in 1959 could be ruled out because my dad's CV in the

Victoria Wellington University yearbooks for 1960 to 1962 showed his highest qualification was a master's degree from Cornell.

This fact alone meant that both the red Doctor of Science and the blue PhD were both fakes. They were designed to work together as a pair because the biography inside the front cover of the red DSc had been manipulated to explain them both:

'After spending a short time at the Thomas More Institute, Montreal, he undertook post-graduate work at Cornell University Ithaca, NY, where he graduated with degrees MS (1958), and PhD (1959).'

Around the date on the DSc document, July 1961, other sources show that my dad was still being truthful about his qualifications. The 1960–61 Victoria University yearbook is just one example. So, the red thesis couldn't have been made on the date inscribed on its cover because there is a lie on its first page. It must have been made later, possibly a lot later. In the absence of a better explanation, I supposed it was probably created at the same time as the fake PhD.

My dad added an unnecessary flourish to his new introductory biography: *'He is married with one son'*, which would have been true if it had been written in July 1961, when my brother was three months old. Was he trying to bolster the case for it having been made on the date he pretended? After 1963, he had both a son and a daughter: me. My dad could conceivably have been playing the part of a man with only one child, his younger, less encumbered self.

Isn't the expression 'one son' a little strange, anyway? Isn't it more natural for the father of one boy to say 'I'm married with a son'? Unless there were, at that moment, already two of us playing somewhere in the house. Would he have felt any discomfort at all if he denied my existence as he typed it?

One child or two, what's the difference? It's not a curse to imagine for once that she isn't there. That she might never be.

What about 'one child', how does that sound? No, no good. No father of a single child would be so indifferent to their sex.

'One son' is better.

A small but significant twist on the life he was living in 1959. A true account still exists as well, of course, in the MSc thesis held by Cornell University library. That version came into being over a year before my brother was conceived and so it doesn't refer to him at all. As nobody needs to know if a doctoral degree candidate has children, my dad put my brother into the story as a superfluous flourish, for his own amusement. Or maybe it's a clue about who the document was intended to fool. A person who would be impressed by the human side of him, by his character, rather than by the science itself. Somebody in a university admin office, perhaps. Or even an interview panel.

What was more difficult to know was whether he had really been awarded a Doctor of Science degree, but later made a fake red book as concrete proof.

My second university librarian, in Wellington, New Zealand, was as helpful as she could be, but apologetic. She couldn't say why there was nothing she could show me anywhere in the library, even though their archive policy was the same as Cornell's. Nineteen sixty-one was a long time ago. There was no other copy of the red thesis. There seemed to be nothing more I could do to prove whether it was a complete fabrication.

The red thesis is noticeably slim and slight, less than half the thickness of its blue counterpart. The blue one has 134 single-sided pages, whereas the red book has only 44. Bearing in mind that the blue book is only an MSc thesis, maybe this is surprising. They are in the same discipline, so they might be expected to be similarly lengthy or succinct.

Inside the blue book, there is a page of acknowledgements expressing gratitude to two professors, to pharmaceutical companies Hoffmann-La Roche and Sigma for the donation of research samples, and for 'the assistance of my wife in the preparation of graphs'. But the red volume acknowledges nobody at all. And from that point on, the red book is completely different from its partner.

This is because the red book is not a thesis at all. It's called: *An application to the University of New Zealand for the degree of Doctor of Science, by Michael Harvey Briggs,* and it's a collection of letters and articles, inexpertly photocopied from journals and from disassembled loose-leaf volumes, then paginated sequentially. It has no introduction, thesis, antithesis or conclusion, and it is in four distinct sections.

The first contains a five-page article about the eye-colour of crabs, published in *Nature* in May 1961, and another five-page article about woodlice collected in the Upper Hutt valley, in New Zealand, published in *The Australian Journal of Biological Sciences.*

The second section is a twelve-page article from *Comparative Biochemistry and Physiology,* about ascorbic acid in the New Zealand cockroach.

The third section is a short letter published in *Nature* in July 1960, proposing a theory of carcinogenesis through the examination of coenzymes in a rat's liver.

The fourth section, made up of a five-page article in *The New Zealand Journal of Geology and Geophysics* and a nine-page article in *Nature* from September 1961, is probably the most surprising. After examining a meteorite that landed in Mokoia, New Zealand, in 1908, and had since been in a local museum, my dad proposes there are compounds inside that were plausibly 'the decomposition products of an extra-terrestrial life-form'.

It's true that great science can be made about the tiny and the apparently trivial. But the papers in this collection are very few and very short, and together, they go nowhere. The fourth section, had the extra-terrestrial point been well-founded, would at the very least have won my dad a Nobel Prize. But clearly it didn't.

My brother has a doctorate but his is in mathematics, not in science. He'd hinted to me that he thought what was in the red thesis was very strange, but like a lot of things about our dad, there'd been no reason for either of us to question why this might be. Now, we had good reason to doubt it all.

There is another, more practical problem with the red thesis. The article from *Comparative Biochemistry and Physiology* was received for publication in September 1961, two months after the red thesis was apparently submitted for assessment. And the version of the article which is inside the red book is a reprint, dated 1962. That alone pushes back the date for the red book's creation to at least a year after the date embossed on the cover.

The red book is indisputably another fake, and not a convincing one.

17

But the question remained: was there ever a real Doctor of Science degree? Doctor of Science degrees are of a higher order than ordinary doctorates and are awarded for truly exceptional contributions to the sum of knowledge. It now seemed doubtful that my dad could have done such a thing, particularly at such a young age. But just because the red DSc thesis had turned out to be counterfeit, that on its own didn't prove the lack of the qualification it pretended to be.

When my dad arrived at Victoria University, it had existed for over fifty years but it had never been an autonomous institution. It was called Victoria University College because it was a college of the University of New Zealand, with no power to award its own degrees. My dad applied for a Doctor of Science degree in July 1961 to the University of New Zealand, and what he handed in was probably very like the bundle of documents in the red thesis. But it can't have been the same because the red thesis has things in it that weren't published at the time.

By early 1961, it had already been decided that the national University of New Zealand would devolve degree-awarding powers to Victoria, with the legal handover taking place at midnight on New Year's Eve of that year. Temporary measures were put into place to cover any applications sent in during the transition, like my dad's. Two examiners would report to the Victoria Senate and decide whether the degree should be awarded, if the candidate had demonstrated 'an original contribution of special excellence to some branch of pure or applied science'.

The university records are confusing because of this handover of power in 1961/62. All that remains regarding my dad's application is an archived file note. Professor George Wald at Harvard University and Professor Ernest Baldwin in London agreed to act as the external examiners. Wald was a biological chemist who would later win the Nobel Prize for physiology. Baldwin was another highly respected scientist, who had written the first textbook about biochemistry as a new scientific discipline. They were each sent copies of my dad's submission, which were delivered in January of 1962.

Their shared opinion is set out in the file note in a single word: 'unfavourable'. The papers were sent back to Victoria in April 1962 and each of the professors was paid the agreed fee of ten guineas. And that, one might think, should have been the end of that.

It's hard to see how it was possible for the university Senate to award a DSc when the submission had been turned down by both examiners. Whoever judged the merit of what my dad had sent in and decided that it was 'an original contribution of special excellence', it wasn't Professors Wald and Baldwin. So something very strange had happened when my dad asked Wellington University for a DSc. I wondered if there were any living witnesses who could remember what it was.

I trawled the archives looking for the co-authors of collaborative papers published between 1959 and 1962. The first few leads were dead ends, which was perhaps not surprising after sixty years. Then I searched the next name on the list: George Barrie Kitto.

G Barrie Kitto had been a twenty-three-year-old student at Victoria University when my dad arrived on campus in 1959.

Born and brought up in Wellington, New Zealand, he'd gone to his local university to study chemistry, then stayed on for an extra year to do a master's degree. By 2020, he'd become emeritus professor of molecular biosciences at the University of Texas in Austin. I contacted him through the university and he quickly responded, saying he'd be delighted to talk to me. He no longer wrote very much because after years of failing sight, he had gone blind.

I phoned Professor Kitto not long after his eighty-third birthday, in the summer of 2021. He still had the New Zealand softness in his voice, despite having lived in the United States since the 1960s. He and his wife moved to America when he took up a graduate post at Brandeis University, Massachusetts, where he completed his doctorate in 1966.

In 1959, Barrie Kitto had been in awe of the new member of the chemistry faculty. He'd always thought that my dad was significantly older, maybe five or six years older than him, when in fact my dad was born only a year before him, in 1935. From the very beginning, my dad projected both intellectual and personal authority. By the time he came to Wellington, he already had a professional reputation, with recent and direct experience at the cutting-edge of scientific research from elsewhere in the world. He brought with him a stylish and pretty wife, who made her own clothes in modern European styles. When my parents had arrived from Britain via America by steamship, the only way to get to New Zealand at the time, it was as if they'd come to this remote part of the globe from the future. Michael Briggs already seemed to be a larger-than-life figure, although still in his mid-twenties.

※ ※ ※

'Call me Barrie, won't you?'

'Thank you, Barrie, yes of course. Tell me, did you meet the other members of the family?'

'Yeah, I met your mum. I'm not sure I met your brother but I remember congratulating your dad when he was born. Your parents didn't get to our wedding in June 1961 because your brother was sick, I think. He was a tiny baby, of course.'

'And did you hear about what happened in 1986, before my dad died?'

'Yeah, I did, that was really sad. The evidence that got into the papers was pretty strong. I thought he'd committed fraud on a pretty big scale.'

'I don't think there's any doubt he did what they said.'

'But I can't understand why he would do it. Do you know why?'

'No, not really. That's one of the things I've been trying to work out.'

'The thing with your dad is he was very driven, what they call a type-A personality. Very full of ideas and not inhibited by anything. But when I knew him, I wouldn't have said he was dishonest or motivated by anything other than the desire to know more.'

'It seems at some point he started pretending to have a doctorate from Cornell.'

'Well, he never said that back then. Not to me. No way. I knew he had a master's from Cornell and that was it. If he did anything like that, it must have been later.'

'What was your relationship with my dad like?'

'I really liked him. I really, really liked him. I got from him the sort of confidence to think anything was possible and that really helped me in my career. I was a kid then, who'd just graduated. And he took me along with him, then we wrote a few papers together. He'd turn up on campus with an idea and he'd say this thing or that thing. Schizophrenia and vitamin deficiencies, maybe. He'd have an idea, then, before you knew it, we were 'off to the races', if you see what I mean. I would never have even applied to Brandeis if it hadn't been for him; I wouldn't have dared. I don't think Brandeis would have looked at me twice if I hadn't had this really unusual, long list of publications. For somebody so young, as young as I was. And that was down to him. We'd been in a huge series of papers in the journal *Nature*, about meteorites. It was nothing to do with my master's at all. We just did it.'

'Barrie, what can you remember about the Doctor of Science degree?'

'That happened sometime in early 1961, the year I got married. I saw your dad one day and he was really happy about something. He said he found out he could get a doctorate by just putting in some papers he'd already written.'

'What did you think about that?'

'Well, I was surprised. I'd never heard of anything like that before. I thought people got DScs for a lifetime's worth of research. Staff in the faculty were surprised too, and annoyed. As time went on, there was some bad feeling about it. That if you could do that you weren't playing the game. It's almost like cheating.'

'Do you think he got the DSc?'

'Yeah, I've always believed so.'

'What happened when it was awarded? Was there a ceremony or a party or something?'

'No, there was nothing. Nobody said anything. Which, now I think about it, was very, very strange.'

* * *

Barrie Kitto remembered that the award of this degree was not celebrated in any way, either at the university itself or in the wider New Zealand scientific community. No congratulations were published in the yearbooks to mark my dad's apparent success. Wellington University curiously failed to advertise its first self-awarded DSc, which was also the first DSc from anywhere to be held by anybody in its science department. The event was marked with silence. My dad was an active member of the Chemistry Society of New Zealand, but its journals also say nothing about it, while several other Doctor of Science degrees awarded to other members were marked with photographs and valedictory editorials. All these awards were made to industry chemists and academics in their forties and fifties for their sustained commitment to the advancement of their discipline. The kind of people one might expect would deserve a DSc.

There is a dark shadow over the award of my dad's DSc degree, which is recorded in just five words in the minutes of a Senate meeting on 29 October 1962. My parents and infant brother had already left New Zealand by then, for Pasadena. In a paper co-written with a NASA colleague in late 1962, my dad describes himself as a member of the faculty at Victoria University, working at Caltech's Jet Propulsion Laboratory in California. This shows that he originally went to the space programme on loan. He would have been expected to go back to Wellington and significantly enhance the university's prestige.

My dad must have known much earlier in the year that he was going on secondment to Caltech JPL. This would have been an incredible opportunity for any scientist, and particularly for one based in a chemistry department in Wellington, New Zealand. It meant that any negotiations about his DSc degree, particularly after the idea was conclusively rebuffed by Wald and Baldwin, were conducted with my dad holding a trump card. His personal success was now so closely tied to the university's advancement that it was in everybody's interests for him to be given what he wanted. He had the potential to put a small New Zealand university onto the world stage in space science – but only if he was willing to come back.

Degrees now fell within the discretion of Victoria University's Senate – they had just been given the power to bypass rejection by Professors Wald and Baldwin, when in previous years it would have been an insurmountable obstacle. If they wished to, they could reward a man who promised to be a trophy for the institution, in exchange for which he should be willing to return. Perhaps the Senate justified its actions by casting the external assessors' opinion as old-world snobbery. Surely Wald and Baldwin had to be wrong if Caltech had made Michael Briggs one of the chosen few on the space programme? It was evidence enough of his talent to justify bending the rules, just a little bit.

Looking back, I think the job at Caltech JPL and the Doctor of Science degree were conjured into existence by the same sleight of hand. If my dad's application to JPL was successful because he told Caltech he was about to be awarded a Doctor of Science degree, and if the Doctor of Science degree was waived through by Victoria University because my dad was of interest to Caltech JPL, then he'd gambled on getting both and had won.

Colleagues in the Victoria chemistry faculty had little choice but to accept that one of the university's highest honorariums was being awarded to a twenty-seven-year-old without even a PhD to his name, but they didn't have to like it. There appears to have been a policy of silence around the decision. A public announcement and a celebration, marking the achievement of the individual and the success of the team, would have been natural. But nothing at all was said.

My dad never went back to Wellington, of course. He found something else he would rather do instead, in Wiltshire. He only ever travelled in one direction: forwards, away from the smoke of burning bridges.

✻ ✻ ✻

After their paths had crossed in New Zealand in the early 1960s, Professor Barrie Kitto went on to become the scientist my dad never was. His decades-long struggle to understand the complex operation of immunotoxins has helped to make HIV a manageable condition instead of a death sentence. When I spoke to him, he was mystified by the idea that research might be faked. Inventing test results was contrary to every scientist's instinct. He remembered my dad as a man whose enthusiasm ignited his own passion for research. You could say my dad changed the course of Barrie Kitto's life in science for the better, even if his influence was inadvertent. Which was a good thing for Professor Kitto, and for humanity.

The young Barrie Kitto learned from my dad that it was possible to shape his own destiny by leaving the small city in the small country where he was born and taking risks. He seized the chance when it came to go to Massachusetts, just as my dad had once set off for Canada, to see if he could make his own luck.

What separated Barrie Kitto from my dad was the difference in their characters. In 1961, Barrie Kitto had similarly stopped believing his native town to be the world but, unlike my dad and Victor Frankenstein, his nature was more than equal to his aspirations.

Emeritus Professor Barrie Kitto died in February 2024. He was eighty-six. He and his wife Binnie had been married for sixty-five years, since the wedding my parents missed in 1961.

18

I've gone round to see my brother, to give him back the blue and red books for safe keeping.

'The world isn't a rational place,' I say to him. 'It's full of inexplicable coincidences. If it hadn't been for some random wild reptiles, we would never have found out what kind of man our dad really was. We'd have assumed forever he really was the man who knew all science.'

'Toads aren't reptiles,' my brother replies. 'They're amphibians. And university registrars aren't usually reptiles either.'

'The point is that if dad hadn't seen the snake eat the toad on the path, we would never have questioned his qualifications. He would've gone back to his office before he resigned from Deakin and got rid of the fakes he'd made.'

'Though why he felt that way about what he saw, or thought he saw, remains a mystery to me.'

'But it doesn't matter why, does it? Maybe it was a real experience, maybe not. Maybe it was a hallucination, or a neurotic overreaction, or even some sort of portentous supernatural event. Who knows? Fate sent a hungry snake into his path, cutting him off from his office. And if he'd gone back, he would either have got rid of the incriminating evidence – these books – or he would have taken them with the rest of his library to Spain. So, we would never have got them.'

'This is true. Apart from the Fate thing you sneaked in there.'

'It can't simply be chance, surely? It's kismet, karma, call it what you like. Because then the sparkly gold lettering on the covers caught the eye of the registrar. And he decided not to throw them away either.'

'This registrar is more magpie than reptile. Or Smaug.'

'On top of that, if the parcel had been posted any earlier and they'd arrived when dad was still alive, he still would have had the opportunity to dispose of them or put them out of harm's way. They still wouldn't have got to us.'

'I don't think we'll ever know what happened to everything else he owned. So – yes.'

'If they'd been sent any later, then they would probably have been lost as well. They'd have arrived at the empty house of a dead man.'

'It is all very surprising, I agree.'

'Surprising! It is a perfect coalescence of chance events.'

'Everything is equally unlikely until it happens, then it just becomes what happened.'

'You still don't think there could be some mysterious power somewhere in the universe. Something that can subtly influence human events?'

'Frankly, I don't.'

I hand the books to him.

'You always knew anyway, didn't you? That Dad's DSc was all nonsense.'

'I wouldn't say exactly that I always knew,' he replies. 'It's not my field. I'm a mathematician. I can't say how good the science might be. Or might have been. It's sixty years old, after all.'

'But you read it and you could see there was pretty much nothing there.'

'Ah, yes. But when I read it before, I thought he had a PhD. So, if the DSc looked a bit inadequate, I thought, well, maybe in science that's normal. But he didn't have a PhD at all. That changes things.'

'Why?'

'Because the so-called DSc is just a small bundle of unrelated papers, without a PhD behind it. So Dad never completed a proper piece of academic research. Something you'd assume he'd done, from his CV. Twice, in fact.'

'There were signs,' I say. 'In hindsight. We shouldn't have been so credulous.'

'It wasn't down to us to work it out,' he says. 'We were just his kids. And dad was churning out – well, is there a nice way of saying it? Content-free research? Or possibly freely applied opinion? He'd been writing like that since before we were born. And a good ten years before he became research director at Schering, of course.'

My brother takes the theses to his office and comes back with a book, *The Handbook of Philosophy*.

'I used to love that book,' I say. 'I loved it because our dad made it.'

'I know you did. But it's rubbish. He was a twenty-two-year-old with a chemistry degree. He got up one day and scribbled something about the whole of philosophy, from Plato to Sartre. Why it was published at all is hard to fathom.'

I take the book and open it.

'I used to think I might find clues in it. About Dad, about what he thought and how he felt.'

My brother snorts.

'Truer than you knew! Look up "Moral Sense", for example.'

I flick through to the Ms.

'It says "Moral Sense, *see Moral Faculty*".'

I flick back a couple of pages.

'"Moral Faculty. The ability to choose between *Right* and *Wrong* actions."'

'So, you can look up the definition of "Right" . . .'

'Which is "the belief that a thing is correct, true, good, preferable, satisfactory, etc". And "Wrong" . . .'

I search through the Ws.

'Ah. Dad's left out "Wrong", after all. There's no "Wrong" in the book.'

'Well, there we are.'

'That's quite a good joke,' I say. 'But it might just be a printer's error, mightn't it?'

'There's a throwaway comment in the introduction about plagiary, which is quite telling. He admits he's ripped off so many other people's books it would be impossible to acknowledge them all. So, he doesn't even try.'

'I can see that's poor. But then again, he was very young. We all did things that we wouldn't do now. What about everything else he wrote, all the science textbooks and the articles? They can't all be no good, can they?'

'He published a lot more than most of his peers but nearly all of it doesn't bear scrutiny. It was autosuggestion: a man who says so much must know what he's talking about.'

'I still don't see what makes you so certain that Dad wasn't brilliant?' I say. 'People thought he was at the time, didn't they?'

'Well, if you can name it, he had an opinion about it, that's for sure. Crab's eyes. Vitamin deficiencies and mental illness. The origin of the solar system. Nutritional problems of manned spaceflight.

The origins of life on Earth. The colouring matter and radio emissions of Jupiter. Martian society. Lunar tektite. Superior galactic communities, whatever they might be. The age of the universe. Gases on Venus. The science fiction novels of H G Wells. Chemicals in moon dust. Robots. The blue haze of Mars. Then there's those carbonaceous chondrites and the Mokoia meteor, of course—'

'Okay, okay.'

'He wrote more sensibly with collaborators, it seems. Your friend Barrie Kitto is a good example.'

'I know you say it's not possible Dad was a "man who knew all science". But if he was young and enthusiastic, and if he had a lot of interests—'

'That's not the point. You can find things out these days, with the internet. On his own, he wrote almost nothing that was original. It's nearly all literature reviews, "in conclusion, more research would be a good idea", that kind of thing. Or it's student workbench stuff.'

'Well, what about the hormone research, though? I saw his series *Oral Contraception* in his study when I was in Spain. It looked like dozens of volumes.'

'It's hard to say now what was in it because most of his books were pulped after the 1986 research scandal. But his series *Oral Contraception* was published by Eden Press. And Eden Press was the pet project of a man very like our dad, called David Horrobin. They shared what you could call a freewheeling attitude to the business of science.'

'Meaning?'

'I'm only saying it wasn't exactly a university press. Dad's books weren't usually handled by mainstream academic publishers.

So there was little or no peer review. Some publishers don't insist on peer review at all. Even some big science publishers. Then bundles of unreviewed papers are often turned into sponsored books at pharmaceutical conferences. They get into circulation, onto shelves, into libraries. Dad was editor of quite a few of those.'

It all sounded like the sort of thing that publishers of pulp fiction novels might do, not science textbooks.

By the late 1960s, my dad was exploiting various unfiltered routes into publication: collections of papers that were really drug company catalogues, and small, uncritical publishing houses outside the scientific mainstream. Producing a lot of books improved his status, and high status led to more and bigger books. As more and more volumes of work by M H Briggs stacked up on the shelves, it became increasingly unlikely that anybody would question the reliability of their source.

'But that's exactly the point, though, isn't it?' I say. 'He didn't keep what he was doing a secret. It's just that nobody seems to have been able to see it. Or maybe it was just unbelievable.'

'It was the 1960s,' my brother says. 'He talked a lot about science and he seemed to have the right credentials. Other men tended to like him. That's probably all that was needed.'

'If you suspected he was a fraud,' I say, 'why didn't you tell me?'

'I was never sure there was anything to tell. Maybe I assumed that's how it always was with people like that. Successful people, I mean. That there's always some exaggeration, some smoke and mirrors.'

'You aren't like that,' I say.

'Well, I'm not successful that way, am I? I wouldn't know how.'

'It's funny that our dad's only son isn't very good at lying.'

He smiles.

'It's not how we do things on Vulcan,' he says. 'But as I've got older, I've learned from experience that the whole truth isn't always helpful. You liked believing our dad was the Wizard of Oz. It was comforting, even after the research scandal, after he was dead. In the back of your mind, he was still the same as he was when you were a little girl. He'd just made a mistake, that's all. But now it turns out he really was the Wizard of Oz. Because he was a just an ordinary man all along. Hiding behind a curtain, pretending. Which is, I think, somehow more interesting.'

After a moment, I break the silence.

'But do you think he knew what he'd done? Did he know that was all he really was?'

'Yes,' my brother says, with a sigh. 'Of course, he bloody did. He must have known at the end that the missing research would be the very least of it, once everybody knew the scientist who was supposed to have done it wasn't there either.'

19

Friday, 26 September 1986

Michael closed his eyes and put his head back against the seat. Lunch had made him sleepy, and the train was moving with a gently rocking tempo.

After a few minutes, the fantasy began again, about the lawyers and the meeting. Although this time it was different. This time he could see it all so much more clearly. The barrister, the grand, book-lined conference room, the afternoon sun.

This time, the barrister was very young and slight, with close-cropped hair, like a boy.

'I hope you've got deep pockets – you're going to need them, for a case like this,' she said.

'Deep enough,' he replied.

'And I hope you've got nothing to hide,' she said.

'I'm used to getting what I want.'

'That wasn't what I asked.' She leaned closer to him across the table. 'Squeaky clean, are you, *Doctor* Briggs? A man of character? I should hope so, with all those fancy letters after your name.'

Michael felt his mouth opening, to say what he had planned. To tell her he was a man of unimpeachable reputation. But no sound came out.

'Because if there is anything. Anything at all you'd rather the world didn't know about you, *Doctor* Briggs, anything disreputable, dishonest or even unwise, then you can be certain that your opponents, your enemies, will find it out.'

The carriage jolted violently, throwing him forward and down, onto his knees. He fell heavily against the seat opposite, taking his breath away.

'And when you get found out, you'll lose,' she said.

The train had stopped abruptly at the platform of a small, intermediate station, beside an empty, white-painted waiting room and a closed ticket office.

'And when you lose, you'll be ruined. The papers will come after you, to destroy you. Financially. Professionally. Personally. And you will never be free of it.'

It was then that he looked up and saw the name of the station. I'm almost there, he thought. The place where I used to live, years ago. With Marion, and the children.

Mist covered the surrounding fields, and a thin ribbon of longer grass and rushes described the line of the brook, stretching away to the land's edge. In that moment, he remembered it all. Just over that hill would be the house. My house. My study. All my books.

'It won't be one war,' she went on. 'It will be war after war, to your annihilation.'

I wonder if I could open the carriage door, step down onto the platform, then close the door behind me, he thought. Perhaps the train would then move away and very soon it would be gone. Perhaps I might watch it disappear, and then I could walk to the end of the platform and over the metal bridge. Through the wooden gate and down to the brook. If I follow the brook, maybe I'll go back there.

The voice continued in his head. 'Then – then, they will drive over your ruins. You will never rest, not even in a grave.'

The train started up again and Michael watched the station pass the window.

'And when the wind blows through and scatters your dust,' – she lifted her hand up to her face and blew gently across her palm – 'there will be absolutely nothing left to show that you were ever there.'

PART 2

NO REASON TO DOUBT

'Seek happiness in tranquillity, and avoid ambition, even if it be only the apparently innocent one of distinguishing yourself in science.'

Victor Frankenstein,
Frankenstein by Mary Shelley

'"Professor Briggs has a very high rank in the medical community ... He's looked upon as a real authority in the field," said Dr Ursula Lachnit-Fixson, head of Schering's hormone research. "We have no reason whatsoever to doubt that his work has been done correctly."'

'The Bogus Work of Professor Briggs' by Brian Deer
Sunday Times, 28 September 1986

20

Until the launch of Primodos by Schering Chemicals as it then was, if a woman needed to know if she was pregnant or not, she could ask a toad. Toads are very adaptable and as opportunities for work as witches' familiars were drying up, they found an opening on the fringes of twentieth-century medicine. The female clawed toad, *Xenopus laevis*, will spawn in sympathy within days if injected with a pregnant woman's urine. She'll always be right and the injection won't kill her. But keeping Delphic laboratories full of toads wasn't a very modern or efficient thing to do, and as synthetics replaced more of the traditional materials of daily life, the toads looked increasingly old-fashioned and anachronistic.

Primodos first went on sale in the UK in 1959. It was handed out to women who had missed one or more periods as it could provide a quick response to the question 'Am I pregnant?' by inducing menstruation, even though there would have been a natural answer, sooner or later. Modern science had intervened to deliver clinical certainty on demand, although with hindsight, it's far from clear how significant the problem was that Primodos had been created to solve, given the potential risks.

Primodos was the direct ancestor of all the oral contraceptives that were about to come onto the market; it was made from the same man-made chemicals as the pill, only in a much larger dose. In the years to come, these hormones would be arranged into scores of different combinations, with each new version of essentially the same product given a new name and a new advertising campaign: Minovlar, Cerazette, Microgynon, Dianette and Yasmin are among its many daughters and granddaughters.

With its catchy slogan: 'A Toad is Slow to Let You Know!', Schering's 1960s advertising campaign for its new drug appeared on posters in health centres and hospitals as well as in full-page advertisements in clinical journals. It featured a toad climbing over a pile of medical textbooks, waving a spindly forefoot in a friendly greeting, and its light-hearted appeal seems to have been aimed at both professionals and patients. It was well known that animals were used for time-consuming and complicated pregnancy testing in laboratories, so the catchphrase was a shorthand way of publicising a mass-market medical innovation. The slow, good-natured toad provided Schering with a suitable mascot for promoting the advantages of Primodos, before *Xenopus* was dispatched to a life of idleness in the brooks from which they came.

Primodos had previously been marketed as a treatment for irregular menstrual bleeding, a less lucrative field of pharmaceutical sales than diagnosis of early pregnancy. This new angle for an existing compound had the potential to reach a bigger market of healthy women wanting information rather than treatment for illness. It originally cost five shillings to the National Health Service, when it wasn't given away for nothing. It was popular with many British GPs, in part because in some areas they received a steady stream of samples from company reps, to keep in a desk drawer.

There were many countries in which Primodos wasn't licensed at all, which is why controversy about the drug has not been worldwide. In the UK, it was relabelled in 1970 with a warning that it should not be used by pregnant women. In 1975, a second warning was added to the label that the drug 'may cause congenital abnormalities'. But if it had been lying around in a desk drawer for a few years, this warning was likely to go unheeded.

Over time, some women began to report what they believed were miscarriages triggered by Primodos, though it was obviously hard to say if this would have happened anyway. Others thought their babies had been born with missing limbs and other congenital difficulties because of it. In a number of developing economies with poorer systems of healthcare, there were rumours that Primodos would induce abortion, particularly if a double dose could be obtained.

A reported correlation between Primodos use, foetal injuries and miscarriages was first made public in a letter from paediatrician Dr Isabel Gal in the journal *Nature* in 1967, over ten years before the drug was removed from sale in the UK. Dr Gal was the first of several scientists to become convinced that there was something badly wrong with Primodos.

Political interest in Primodos has waxed and waned over the decades, despite the concerns of a number of prominent people. If there had been a scandal, then it never seemed to gain any traction. The alleged victims and campaigners, and their supporters in Parliament, did their best to keep the spotlight on the Primodos affair. But still, little or nothing was done.

In 2014, a review by the Medicines and Healthcare Products Regulatory Agency found the evidence that Primodos caused foetal harm to be inconclusive. In October 2017, an Expert Working Group (EWG) was asked to consider whether the chemicals in

Primodos – norethisterone or ethinylestradiol – could or would cause malformations. They saw a lot of paperwork, including heavily redacted and confidential reports sent to them by Schering, some of which dated back to the 1960s. They were also given recent research using animal models that appeared to show a new biological mechanism for a causal connection. The EWG concluded that the evidence did not show that Primodos was at fault. The EWG agreed that the restriction on Primodos use which should have stopped it from being given to pregnant women did not get through to some GPs, who carried on using it as a pregnancy test when it was known to be a risk.

Disquiet both inside and outside Parliament led Prime Minister Theresa May to appoint Baroness Cumberlege to carry out the medicines review. In 2020, she used the expression 'avoidable harm' to describe the position of the people affected. Primodos briefly became newsworthy again a few months later, when Health Secretary Matt Hancock said there has been 'a scandal'. He apologised for the harm and for the time it has taken for the Primodos victims' voices to be heard, but still nothing was said about compensation.

Post-Cumberlege, the Conservative government did nothing, perhaps in deference to the ongoing court proceedings.

21

I want to talk in particular about Primodos. As several colleagues have said, very vulnerable women went to their GP for help, because they thought they might be pregnant. They were myriad different ages, from myriad different parts of the country and certainly from different economic backgrounds. This touched everyone. That GP, in an NHS GP's surgery, pulled open a drawer, gave them some tablets and said, 'This will tell you whether you are pregnant'—no advice, no concerns, no documentation . . . Some had miscarriages, some were told to abort the child and some went on to have children with abnormalities that were frightening then and today. The types of disabilities were similar to those of thalidomide, and one might have thought that we would have learned the lesson of thalidomide . . . But no—we have not learned those lessons . . . People ask me why GPs were doing this. It was because drugs company salespeople were going into the GP surgeries and pushing their product at the doctors, promoting it so they could earn more and more money . . . Some people—particularly those affected by Primodos—will pass away. But we will not go away. We will go on and on and on about it in this House until compensation is provided to our constituents, and that is the right thing to do.

Sir Mike Penning, Conservative MP for Hemel Hempstead

Hansard, 3 February 2022

In January 1975, my constituent, Nan, was prescribed two Primodos tablets as a pregnancy test by her doctor. It was subsequently confirmed that at that time she was about seven or eight weeks pregnant. There is considerable evidence indicating that those women who took the drug, prescribed by their GPs, and were pregnant at the time, gave birth to babies with serious birth defects, including deformities and disabilities, missing limbs, cleft palates, brain damage and damage to internal organs. In some cases, the women miscarried or had stillbirths.

At the time, in 1975, Primodos had already been banned for use as a pregnancy test for five years in Norway and Sweden. When my constituent's daughter, Michelle, was born in August 1975, it was immediately discovered that she had a hole in her diaphragm, which had allowed her bowel and spleen, part of her liver and kidney to be forced into her chest cavity, crushing her lung. Michelle was not expected to live, but thanks to the skills of our NHS she survived and is now 46 years of age. Throughout her life, Michelle has endured numerous operations and surgeries and long, long periods of hospitalisation, has suffered severe health issues, including breathing difficulties, a weakened immune system, numerous bowel obstructions and inflammatory bowel infections, and has been unable to conceive children. The effects of those debilitating physical and psychological medical and extremely challenging health conditions suffered by Michelle for the last 46 years just cannot be adequately described in words.

Allan Dorans, SNP MP for Ayr, Carrick and Cummock

Hansard, 3 February 2022

22

As I read more about the strange history of Primodos, I saw glimpses of my dad, like archaeological finds: a letter here, a name there, another picture, like a pot shard or a belt buckle sticking out of the mud. One such fragment was his nine-minute interview in the programme *The Primodos Affair*, which nobody is allowed to see. Another was his connection with Dr Isabel Gal, who had first pointed the finger of blame. It turned out that she and my dad had met more than once, in 1967.

In a speech in the 1980s to the association of Primodos families, Isabel Gal described being invited to a meeting at a restaurant shortly after her concerns were published in *Nature*. The meeting was with my dad, as research director of Schering UK, medical director Alan Pitchford and Ursula Lachnit, the most senior scientist at international Schering AG. Strangely, Dr Lachnit's presence bookends the final twenty years of my dad's life, beginning at this meeting with Isabel Gal and ending when she told the *Sunday Times* in 1986 that she knew of no reason to doubt his research.

Dr Gal said my dad had gone to see her some time before the lunch and had asked to take away some of her patient records and notes. This was the first inkling she had that taking action about what she had seen in her neonatal clinic would bring her into conflict with powerful forces. This lunch meeting appears to be the start of a strategy on the part of the three executives to protect sales of the product and the company's reputation by either silencing or discrediting Isabel Gal.

Dr Gal was unreliable in the eyes of the drug producers and regulators, but she was not silenced. Despite her clinical credentials, she was sidelined then ignored, so she lent her support to the Primodos campaigners, who were fighting a system that allied itself with Schering against them. It's hard not to think that Isabel Gal's personal characteristics made her easier to exclude from the discussion, once she'd been labelled as a troublemaker: she was female and she was a Jewish Hungarian refugee who had survived the Auschwitz concentration camp.

Archives show that the government's senior medical safety officer, Dr William Inman, wrote letters to my dad implying that they were on the same side in a battle to prevent 'medico-legal problems'. In 1975, Inman said in correspondence with Schering that Dr Gal was 'a rather sad little person', while at the same time admitting that 'we are defenceless in the matter of the eight-year delay' since the publication of her letter. All the while, Primodos remained on the market. Inman later admitted destroying files of data about the incidence of miscarriage and malformation in the Primodos years, later explaining privately to Schering that he'd done this because of 'the risk of individual legal claims'.

Dr Gal didn't say where it was that they went for lunch that day. A favourite haunt of my dad's around that time was the revolving restaurant above the Post Office Tower. I went there with him when I was about five years old and my brother seven. My dad was attracted to novelty more than most children are, so he needed little excuse to go to restaurants that moved or floated, and he may well have eaten at the Top of the Tower every time he'd been in London since its opening. I remember watching the curving line where the fixed carpet outside the lift met a steady waltz of revolving tables, chairs, diners and waiters, and worrying about having to jump over it to get out.

The Top of the Tower went round twice in the time it would take to eat a three-course lunch. More than enough time for my dad to explain to Dr Gal that her fears about Primodos were unfounded, as the Houses of Parliament and St Paul's Cathedral processed slowly past. If Dr Gal felt she'd travelled a great distance with my dad only to leave through the same door, I have a lot of reasons to sympathise.

23

By the end of the Primodos story's first half-century, the original focus on the drug itself had been lost in a repeating cycle of unsatisfactory or disputed investigations and public inquiries. Cumberlege had become the latest in that line and had given some comfort to the people affected by Primodos by recommending that their voices be heard and a compensation scheme put in place for them. However, the inquiry had been given no power to find fault or to force the government to do anything at all about its recommendations.

The debate had gone round and round like the Top of the Tower, with one side saying that Primodos had caused foetal harm and the other saying it hadn't, for over five decades – but unlike the Top of the Tower, it showed no sign of stopping.

Over the years, my dad's involvement had even been discussed in Parliament. In a debate in the House of Commons in 2014, Yasmin Qureshi MP openly accused my dad of deliberately engineering the collapse of the court case against Schering in 1982 by switching sides.

'Another person I want to allude to is Professor Briggs,' she'd said. 'It is important to explain to the House that the damage claims brought by the victims were discontinued in the 1980s because some of the medical witnesses defected to the defendants, Schering Chemicals, so the case had to be withdrawn. Some of the victims say that the so-called experts who went over to the Schering side had an interesting story. One of those was Professor Briggs.'

Yasmin Qureshi implied that my dad had taken his 'interesting story' to the plaintiff's side, though it's hard to imagine why he would ever have considered speaking out against the company, as she believed that he had. He had a close working relationship with Schering going back to the 1960s. He'd taken part in what could be interpreted as a strategy to neutralise Dr Gal's concerns about Primodos harm, in his then-capacity as regional head of research for the manufacturer of the drug she thought should be banned, in the country where she'd blown the whistle. Nearly twenty years later, when Ursula Lachnit professed confidence to the *Sunday Times* that my dad's work was reliable, the work she was talking about was being funded, at least in part, by Schering. Simple logic would say my dad would have been likely to stand with Schering. But I don't think logic alone would necessarily be a reliable predictor of my dad's behaviour in this situation.

My dad was opinionated and frequently contrary. By 1982, he had a reputation as an expert and an authoritative voice in academic science. He liked to argue, when often he had no real preference either way. Being perceived as Schering's natural gun for hire might also have offended his sensibilities. It's possible he persuaded himself, for a while, that he could carry the case against Primodos over the line, if he'd wanted to do it.

We'll never know what the 'interesting story' was. But the collapse of the Primodos trial in 1982 became a matter of record. At least they had a sympathetic judge, who put a stay on the case to give the plaintiffs time to get the scientific evidence they needed.

If Yasmin Qureshi was right, then something had changed my dad's mind. I wonder if in the process of preparing the case against Primodos he'd had a sudden dose of reality: that his expert persona was really just a mirage. Expert witnesses are cross-examined, often at great length, to undermine the foundations of their opinion. Their CVs are scrutinised and their views are raked over for idiosyncrasies and flaws. He might have decided that the risk of public exposure would be very high, too high, if he'd picked this particular fight with Schering.

24

'It is a bit upsetting, that my own father could have sat there typing and pretended I wasn't there, that his second child never existed.'

'Do you mean the "married with one son" business?' my brother asks.

'I do. He denied me.'

'A bit extreme. Not to mention grandiose. Why take it personally?'

'Because it is personal'.

'I don't agree with that interpretation. It's illogical.'

'Well, Spock, you would say that.'

'You'll find a lot of that kind of thing in a book he liked, *Mathematical Games* by Martin Gardner. What you thought was a natural thing to say, "married with one child", would have been an untrue statement after you were born. A lie, I suppose you'd call it. But "married with one son" is not. It's just not a comprehensive account of his status as a parent, because he had a daughter as well.'

'That's crazy.'

'Makes perfect sense to me. But I don't import intentions to actions from feelings. It's just logical wordplay. Which appealed to him.'

'I suppose there's some comfort in that.'

My brother shrugs.

'If you say so.'

'I've been thinking about the houses again,' I say. 'Do you remember us moving house, from Chippenham to Burgess Hill?'

'Not precisely,' he says. 'I was about five or six at the time. But I remember watching the World Cup final in the new house, so it must have been the first half of 1966.'

'Did you watch it with Dad?'

'No. I don't think he was there.'

'And Mum was still sick.'

'Yes, though she'd recovered enough to be at home a bit more.'

'Can you remember when she first got ill?'

'I'm not sure. I think I can but it's mixed up with what I've been told. Mum was on her own with us, at the house in Chippenham. You were sleeping next to her and when she tried to get out of bed, she collapsed. Then they found out her bones were dissolving. The Burgess Hill house was all on one level because she couldn't really walk.'

'Mum was pregnant with me when they got the house in Chippenham. She always said they came back from California because it was too expensive to have a baby in America.'

'Well, that could have been true,' my brother says. 'But it's a funny reason to come back to England. I always thought Mum wanted to stay in Pasadena. Or the alternative was going back to New Zealand. There's a lot of gaps, aren't there? We'll never know it all. And it's too late to find out now everyone's dead. Though it hardly matters, does it? The past isn't real, really, anyway.'

'I'm just trying to get it clear in my head,' I say. 'If I was born in October 1963, in Wiltshire. Dad got a new job there doing something or other. Research with animals?'

'I do remember animals,' my brother says. 'Particularly the strange cow, as I said. But not the job. I was pre-school age, after all.'

'Then it was sometime between 1964 and 1966 that Mum nearly died. Then Dad got another job, at Schering Chemicals in Burgess Hill.'

'That's correct,' he says.

'Though why either of those last two things happened,' I say, 'I have no idea.'

25

September 1964, Chippenham, Wiltshire

Michael switched off the ignition, then he stayed in the driving seat, looking through the windscreen towards the glass wall that separated the living room from the drive. Marion was kneeling on the floor with her full skirt spread out around her, not quite covering her bare legs and feet. She was smiling at the back of the baby's head, and from the shape of her mouth he could see she was making gentle sounds, encouraging the child back to the safety of a close embrace. The baby's face was turned away from her, hot-red and screaming soundlessly. Her woollen legs flexed on her mother's thigh; her knitted dress twisted up above the puffed-out seat of her tights and her fat arms thrashed hard with a repetitive momentum. She strained with a free hand towards a desired object, a metal truck belonging to her brother, but it remained out of reach where it had rolled and stopped against the edge of the rug. The boy lay on his front playing alone, absorbed in the task of connecting bricks into larger shapes according to an intricate and evolving design. The whole scene, with its modern domestic frame, its backdrop of soft lamps and sparse furniture, and with the distant promise of open-plan dining beyond, looked to Michael like an artfully devised advertisement for an expensive product he no longer wanted to buy.

✻ ✻ ✻

They'd bought the house on the same day they'd seen it, just over a year before. The estate agent had arrived before them and was already opening the front door with several keys.

'You'll have seen from the brochure that it's new, of course. In what I've called the ranch-style: open-plan, single-storey. Continental living. All the mod cons.'

With their evenly tanned faces and ultra-bright summer clothes, the couple had appeared out of a chilly autumnal fog as if they'd travelled back in time rather than across the Atlantic. He'd taken an instant dislike to the man when he'd met him the day before because his directness seemed deliberately rude, particularly in one so young. But the agent's attitude had changed when he realised that the man and his heavily pregnant wife were planning to buy a large house for cash, with American dollars.

'There's teak parquet throughout, ducted underfloor heating everywhere, four beds, a library, a study, a formal dining room with kitchen access. Quite beautiful, don't you think? On the market at £4,000, though there may be room for negotiation, for the right buyer.'

Michael acknowledged the point without speaking and moved away down a long corridor towards the bedrooms, leaving Marion in the vestibule. She opened and closed the hall cupboard, which, like the rest of the house, was empty.

'When are you expecting the new arrival?'

She smiled. 'Early October, so the midwife says.'

Marion looked down, resting her hands on the front of her cotton dress, where the matching jacket no longer buttoned closed.

'Dr Briggs told me yesterday that you two have been all over the world in the last few years.'

'Yes, that's true,' Marion said. 'But Michael's not a doctor. He's a science teacher. Doctor is just an honorary thing, for some papers he wrote, I think. We went to Canada five years ago and got married: he had to get out of Liverpool so he didn't get called up. Then Michael had a thing in New York State, then another one in New Zealand after that.'

'He said you're back here from California, that he's been working on something to do with space rockets?'

'It's an amazing place. But it turned out the job was just temporary. So, he decided – well, we decided – it was time to come home. To settle down.'

'Where is he working now?'

'Corsham, not far from here. This time it's something to do with animal feed, but the government is involved somehow. I'm not entirely sure.'

'Do you have other children?'

'A boy,' Marion said. 'He's two. He's with my mother today.'

'Shall we take a look at the kitchen?'

'If you like. But I'm afraid I'm useless at cooking. Michael was quite surprised when he found out I could only make stuffed peppers, and them not very well.'

She opened the built-in oven and looked inside.

'I was in the rag trade when I met Michael, after I left school. I'd been in digs, so I never had a kitchen. I ate out.'

* * *

As he took out his key and opened the front door, Michael could hear his wife singing.

He'd been gone this time for only one night, at a conference. He'd given a short paper, which wasn't very taxing, just a summary of what he'd been doing for the past year. When he walked back to his seat, he'd smiled at a woman as he passed and she'd smiled back. It was only later that evening, after they'd met again, that he knew everything could be different.

26

'Have you seen the film *Catch Me If You Can?*' I ask my brother. 'I watched it last night.'

'I can see already where this is going,' he replies.

A few months had passed, during which I'd found little more in the way of evidence connecting my dad with the Primodos affair. But I wondered if studying other people like him might help to explain his motivation.

'There are some obvious parallels though, aren't there? Between the character of Frank Abagnale and our dad,' I say. 'Frank Abagnale moves around all the time, to avoid detection. Dad always travelled a lot too, more than most other people, particularly for the time. What if he spent his whole life moving for a reason. And it was only when he stopped moving, in Australia at Deakin, or in any event when he failed to move quickly enough, that he got caught out.'

'Equally, though, shifting from job to job and country to country has practical advantages,' my brother says. 'He was exploiting fresh opportunities, putting himself in new situations. You could say he was just making both personal and evolutionary gains.'

'But that also meant he could take advantage of people who didn't know him. People who had no experience from which they could judge his actions and his motives. Most people are very trusting.'

'Maybe,' my brother says. 'I'm just saying that you can look at it several ways. If human beings had stayed in one place, then our species would have got quite literally nowhere.'

'Abagnale dresses himself up and pretends to be what he's not. As an airline pilot, for example. Isn't forging a doctoral thesis just a version of that?'

'I suppose that depends on why it's done,' he says. 'I think Abagnale gets two main rewards from pretending to be a pilot. He gets money, but more than that, he gets a thrill out of fooling people, out of tricking them then running away. I think Dad wanted something much deeper than that. I think he wanted to be recognised for his cleverness. But he was frustrated by the obstacles he thought were put in his way.'

'What particularly, do you think?' I ask.

'Oh, he probably thought formal qualifications were unnecessary bureaucracy in his case. I think he had a chip on his shoulder, too. He didn't go to Oxbridge. He grew up in a grotty little house in north Manchester. If anything, Frank Abagnale was the more stable character out of the two of them. Frank Abagnale didn't really want to be a pilot. He wanted people to think he was a pilot, which is different.'

'Dad had a low threshold for boredom, which was part of Abagnale's problem too,' I say. 'Dad stepped up a bit further each time he moved, which would have been exciting. Repeatedly re-experiencing intense feelings of success would have been quite addictive. He could be charming, he could blend in, socially. He used intellectual fireworks as a distraction, to stop people scrutinising what he was really doing.'

'Until he couldn't,' my brother says.

'True. Only for so long. The dishonesty had to catch up with him. When I was small, I saw him as such a big man, full of knowledge and confidence. But now I know he was living a lie, what we were looking at was really just a fragile shell he'd created. He had an inflated sense of himself, which probably made him hypersensitive to humiliation when he came under pressure. He could be rigid and legalistic when he felt threatened, which is a kind of suppressed violence. That seems to have happened several times, over the years.'

'Maybe he could have found peace, eventually. If only he'd got what he wanted.' My brother looks away and I wonder if the subject is making him emotional.

'So, what was it you think he wanted?' I ask him.

'Oh, self-respect. Contentment. Some shit like that. How should I know?'

27

September 1964, Chippenham, Wiltshire

Michael took off his jacket and tie, and lay down on the settee, pushing off his shoes onto the floor.

'*There I'll settle down, beneath the palms, in someone's arms, in Pasadena—*'

'For Christ's sake, Marion, stop singing that stupid song. I've got a headache,' he said.

His wife settled the baby against her side, then she moved behind him, bending down to kiss his forehead.

'I saw the new lady next door, today at the post office. She said they'd look in later. She asked us to theirs but there's nobody to sit the children.'

'Couldn't you put them off?'

'Oh, Michael, I know and I'm sorry, but can't you just try? They'll be our neighbours and we don't know anybody here. They won't stay long. I said to come in for drinks in an hour.'

* * *

The man praised Michael for his evident good taste, then Marion took him on a tour of the house. The woman watched them go, then leaned back on the settee and found a pack of cigarettes. Michael pulled out a cardboard matchbook, then remembered the phone number written on the inside fold. He tore out a match and struck it, offering the flame inside his palms.

'Marion's doing a beautiful job with the kids, isn't she? I think she's a natural. Not like me.'

The woman continued to lean towards Michael, breathing the smoke up into her nostrils in a steady stream.

'She's the creative type,' he said. 'It's extraordinary to watch sometimes, she seems to get on with them like equals, almost like they're real people. She can spend hours with them, playing with bits of plastic, sticking their fingers in paint.'

'I couldn't do it,' she said. 'It would bore the pants off me. We're not having any.'

She watched Michael to see what he'd do, but he gave her no visible response.

'He'd have wanted them,' she went on. 'But as I said, it's not him that has to have them and look after them, is it?'

She picked a small flake of tobacco from her lower lip with her fingernail.

'Everybody was surprised when we got married, and none of them more than me. He kept asking and I suppose he caught me at a weak moment. It's nice because he'd do anything for me, but we're chalk and cheese, really.'

Michael's attention had wandered. He could no longer be bothered to feign interest. Not for long enough to make any of this worthwhile.

'So anyway,' she said. 'How did you meet?'

'Oh, the usual way. At a dance. At the university. She came with some of the girls from work.'

'And it was love at first sight, was it?'

A passing thought brought with it an image from the past. A dark cinema, *The Incredible Shrinking Man*. Being suddenly aware of her warm presence in the seat beside him. On the screen,

Scott and Louise lying together on the front deck of a small motorboat, kissing. Before the chemical cloud came. He pushed it quickly out of his mind.

'Oh, no – not at all. We went to the pictures, spent a bit of time together. Found out we had this and that in common.'

'And you're a scientist.'

'Yes. Not the mad kind. I'm a chemist. A biochemist.'

'And you were working in America, before you came back here?'

'On the space programme.'

'It must feel like a bit of a comedown for you. From America to boring old GB.'

He moved away, sliding open the door to the garden.

'I'd love to go to America. I passed the eleven plus, went to the girls' grammar. I used to love science, but I didn't do anything with it at the time.'

He stepped outside and she followed him.

'Marion tells me you're now in the animal feed business?'

Michael paused without turning round.

'Animal nutrition. Yes. I am.'

'I always thought cows ate grass!' Marion appeared around the side of the house and stepped onto the patio with the man close behind her. 'And nobody has to make that,' she said. 'Except Mother Nature, I suppose. But what do I know?'

'I'm sure it's very interesting,' said the woman, 'and nothing's more important than the food we eat, is it?'

'So, what's involved in that then?' the man said.

'It's vitamins. Vitamins, minerals, hormones, exact quantities can mean life or death for everything organic. For all of us, not just farm animals. Most people don't realise even vitamins can kill you.'

'That's fascinating, isn't it? My husband's in retail.'

'I'm a regional manager, for WH Smiths. Where did you say you worked again, Michael?'

'Smiths is great,' said Marion. 'I really missed it when we were abroad.'

'Actually, I didn't say where I worked,' Michael said, 'but it's a few miles from here, in Corsham. At Analytical Laboratories.'

'Corsham?' The man looked at Michael more closely. 'Don't people say there's some funny business going on in Corsham? In the old mine workings?'

'I wouldn't listen to people if I were you,' Michael said. 'I haven't heard anything.'

'They say it's to do with the Russians or something.'

'Well, if I see anybody near the office with snow on their boots I'll be sure to let you know.'

'Do you think you'll work, Marion?' the woman said. 'When the children are bigger? I'd love to work but, as I was saying to Michael, I can't find anything that's worth all the bother.'

While the others carried on talking, Michael drifted back to the previous evening.

He had watched her all the way through dinner from the other side of the room. And she'd looked up now and then to show him that she knew it.

As the delegates trickled out of the dining room, she made her way towards him. She'd stopped to chat a little, or touch, or laugh, but each time she brought her gaze back to his.

'You look bored,' she'd said, eventually sliding into the empty chair next to him.

Her skirt rode up over her knees as she sat down, to the top of a stocking.

'Let's get out of here,' he'd replied.

'Well, first, let me put my proposition. Then you can put yours.'

'Go ahead,' he said.

'I've been asked to tell you there's a job coming up soon we think will interest you, in pharmaceuticals.'

He left her room at dawn, then he'd lain on the bed he hadn't slept in. He'd discovered there were previously unexplored potentialities, in other clandestine lives he could be living. He found himself inclined to exploit them all.

28

'You know we talked about Mum being ill?'

'I've spoken to you several times since,' my brother says. 'But, yes, I remember.'

'I've done some research, about the causes of hypercalcaemia,' I tell him.

'Are there many known causes?' he asks. 'We were always told it was impossible to explain. A one in a million, unexplained illness.'

'Well, it would be one in a million, if it really was unexplained. But there are two quite common reasons for life-threatening hypercalcaemia.'

'I know they said it wasn't a parathyroid tumour, quite early on,' he says. 'Mum had throat surgery in the first few days but that wasn't it.'

'That's the most likely, top of the list. But the second most likely is much harder to detect. It's vitamin overdose, specifically overdosing on vitamin D. Either accidental or deliberate.'

'So, she could have caused it herself?'

'Or somebody else could. Somebody with scientific knowledge, perhaps a biochemist, one with a special interest in toxins.'

'We do know somebody like that, of course. Though it turns out now that he lacked the higher qualifications to be a bona fide evil genius. Are you accusing our dad of attempted murder?'

'I'm just saying it's possible, that's all. I think Dad worked for a couple of years in animal nutrition, between JPL and Schering.

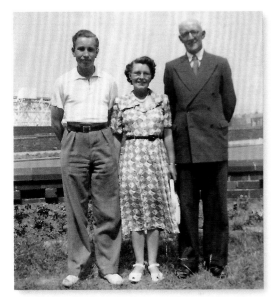
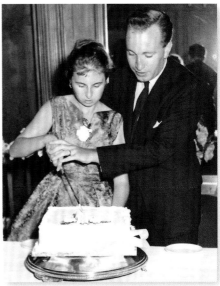
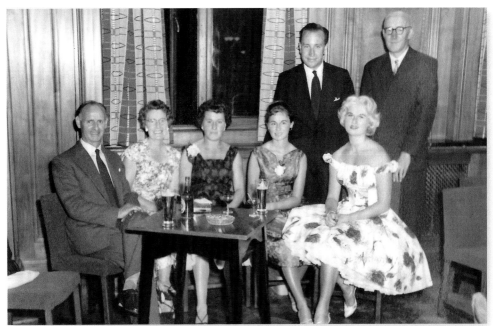

Above left: My dad Michael with his parents, Harry and Flo, on holiday in Blackpool in 1953.

Above right: Their sudden escape to Canada in 1957 had cheated my mother of a bridal photo album, so an event was staged, including this traditional shot of the happy couple cutting the cake.

Below: My dad can be seen standing second from right, alongside his father. In front of my dad, my mother Marion is seated with her parents Jack and Elsie and her younger sister Bebe. It is 1960 and my parents are on a rare visit to Liverpool, England for their 'wedding', when they had in fact been married for nearly three years.

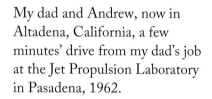

My dad and my brother Andrew in Upper Hutt, Wellington, 1962.

My dad and Andrew, now in Altadena, California, a few minutes' drive from my dad's job at the Jet Propulsion Laboratory in Pasadena, 1962.

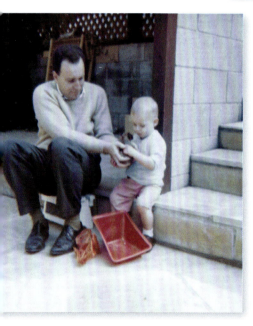

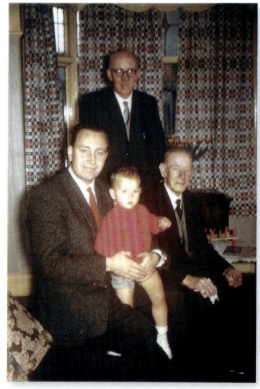

Four generations in one photo, 1963.

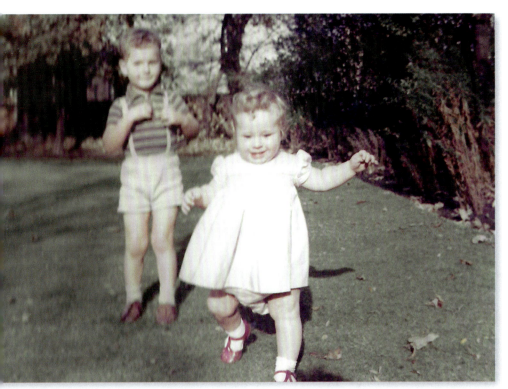

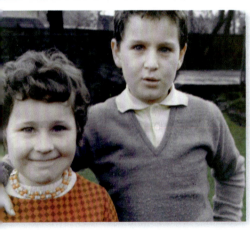

Above: Andrew and me, playing in the garden of our family home in Chippenham, Wiltshire, 1965.

Below left and right: As we grew older, Andrew and I kept each other company. Here, pictured in our Nanna's garden in Manchester in 1969.

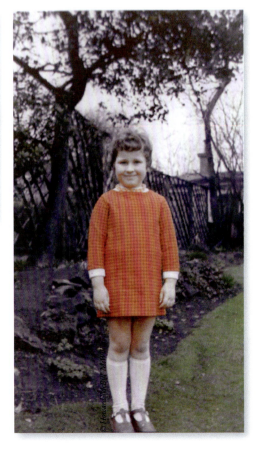

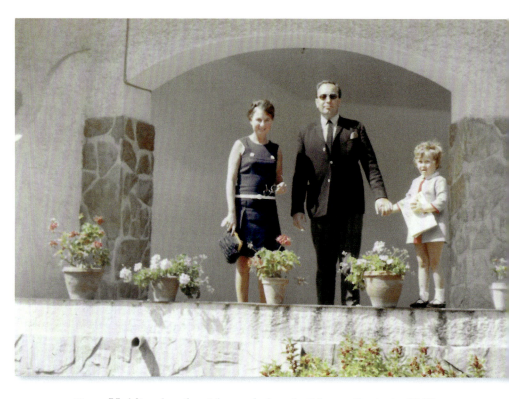

Above: Holding hands with my dad on holiday to Spain in 1968.

Below: My dad again, on the same holiday in Torremolinos in 1968. Eighteen years after this picture was taken, he died only a mile or two away.

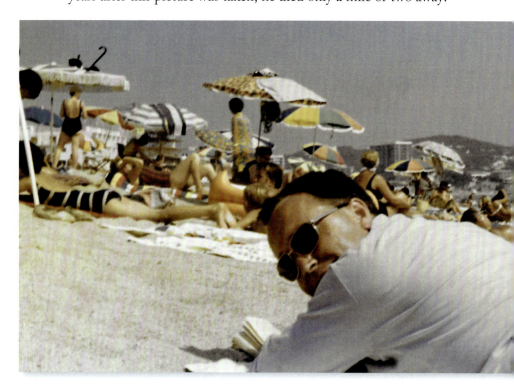

So he'd have had easy access to industrial food additives, if he'd needed them.'

'Oh, I wouldn't disagree it's quite possible,' he says. 'I don't deny that. I think he had a motive, as well. They weren't getting on too well by the time they came back to England, I don't think.'

'And it was much harder in those days to get a divorce', I say. 'He told me once that the best way to poison someone was with something you'd expect to find anyway, in the body. So it's unlikely to be detected at a post-mortem. Not the sort of thing that most parents say to their children, but you know what he was like.'

'He'd probably have thought poisoning was the more attractive option anyway, to be frank. The thing with Dad was that . . . well, he did seem to see other people as either useful or expendable.'

29

September 1964, Chippenham, Wiltshire

Michael was reading when Marion came to bed. She slipped out of her dress and her underwear behind the open wardrobe door, so he saw only a brief outline of her body before she pulled her nightdress over her head. She was still slight but now he saw her as shapeless, somehow blurred. She brushed her hair for a while at the dressing table. As she slid her feet under the bedclothes and curled herself under his arm, he knew he no longer wanted her and never would. In fact, he hated her and would do anything to get away. He used to think of her as a lucky charm. But as far as this charm was concerned, its luck had run out.

For a while, Michael was at home every night and got into a regular morning routine, taking breakfast to the bedroom on a tray. When the next conference came around, he kissed her before he left and said he would be back in a few days, by the weekend. The baby was next to her, peaceful at last, and the gesture seemed to Marion to be a hopeful sign, romantic and kind. She could no longer remember when she hadn't felt tired, so she'd been grateful for the extra help Michael has been able to give her over the last few weeks. As she got dizzier and more disorientated, she wondered if she should see the doctor, but Michael had been reassuring. She was worrying unnecessarily. All young mothers are tired.

Michael had been gone for a couple of hours when Marion woke again. Her pulse was racing and she was soaked with sweat. She tried to get out of bed but was unable to sit upright. It felt for a moment like being on a little boat, rolling with the waves.

I stirred in my sleep on the blanket beside her but did not wake. Mum called out to my brother. After a minute, he appeared in the doorway, rubbing his eyes, still in his pyjamas.

'Can you – help Mummy, sweetheart?' she said. 'I'm not sure I can get out of bed today.'

My brother came to stand at her side. She pushed herself up into a sitting position by leaning on his shoulder. She closed her eyes as the room began to spin.

'That's a good boy, a really, really good boy. Can you sit with your sister now, while Mummy goes to the bathroom?'

Mum stood unsteadily and walked only a few steps towards the door before her legs gave way and she fell. On the floor, she tasted bile in her mouth, and blood.

'Mummy, are you sick?'

She tried to push herself up. She was shaking, her strength all gone.

'Can I have your juice?'

My brother reached for the half-empty glass on the bedside table.

'No! Don't do that, please don't do that!'

He pulled his hand back quickly from the glass and stared at her.

'I'm sorry, I'm sorry. I think the juice might not taste very nice. And I'm not very well, that's all. But I'm alright. I really will be alright, I promise.'

She vomited again, and then she blacked out.

30

Late 1965, Burgess Hill, Sussex

Michael drove to the offices of Schering Chemicals UK, in its purpose-built compound, landscaped into the ring road on the outskirts of the town. In a large conference room, four men and a woman sat along the far side of the table.

'Dr Briggs?'

He might explain about that, he thought, once he had the job.

'Please, call me Michael.'

'Of course. Welcome. You'll be interviewed by our heads of manufacturing and marketing, a representative of the German parent company, by me of course, on behalf of laboratory R&D, and our clinical lead.'

The clinical lead looked up and smiled. She was small and slight, with close-cropped hair like a boy.

'If I can briefly introduce the candidate before we start the interview.'

The panel members turned over a few typed pages and the clinical lead began taking notes.

'As you see from Michael's application, he has certainly had, for a man of his age, a very varied career. For the last couple of years, he's been at Analytical Labs, dealing with various projects. Before that, he was at Caltech, working on a Mars probe. And before that, he was a senior lecturer in New Zealand. So, perhaps to start – why the move into hormonal pharmaceuticals and why Schering?'

Michael took his time, laying out his credentials, steadily revealing an intellectual path that led naturally to that very point. His doctoral research at Cornell was the springing-off point for a career in organic chemistry. JPL had been an unmissable, but time-limited, experience. The job at Analytical Laboratories in Wiltshire was interesting enough, but not a career destination.

'And that brings me on to a special, personal requirement,' he said.

He paused, preparing the effect.

'My wife, Marion, became very seriously ill some time ago and I've been told she is unlikely to survive.'

The chairman shifted uncomfortably in his seat.

'If I'm offered the post, I can only take it if my family, my children, can be nearby. So, if I have to be, I can be both Mum and Dad to them.'

'I doubt that would be a problem, Michael. There would be a relocation package as well as other benefits, for the right candidate.'

The chairman looked round to the other panel members.

'I think that's all we need,' he said. 'Come with me. I'll hand you over to my secretary and she can show you around.'

The interview had gone even better than expected. Circumstances were coalescing in his favour, with a little influence from other interested parties, and his star seemed to be rising again.

The tour took in the clinical and marketing departments, followed by the research and development laboratories, a rotation as colourful and various as Disneyland's Small World boat ride. He began committing to memory everything he heard about the hormone trade, which was soon to be his new area of expertise. They were selling innovations for modern life: tiny pills that guaranteed a fulfilling sex life and a small, happy family. There were brightly coloured posters everywhere. Unlike medicines for illness, nobody had to take any of these drugs if they didn't want them. They needed to be attractive, like washing powders, lipsticks and perfumes. Sisterly Minovlar, Primovlar, and Primodos were only there to make life better.

As Michael prepared to leave, the panel chairman caught up with him and they fell into step as he walked towards the lift.

'Once we've been through all the formalities, I'm sure we'll have some good news for you very soon.'

'I hope so,' Michael said.

'We can talk then about the job, the opportunities for Schering in the marketplace, both here and for Berlin HQ. And Schering's challenges, of course. We have some decisions to make about Primodos. Some fresh eyes on that would be helpful. But that's for another day, once you're on board. I'll come back down to reception with you.'

For a few moments they stood side by side, waiting.

'Tell me if I'm prying but can you tell me what's the matter with your wife?'

'She has severe hypercalcaemia. It came on very suddenly, while I was away on business,' Michael said. 'That was over a year ago, but it's still not under control. Not responding to the standard treatments.'

'They looked at her parathyroid I assume?'

'Oh yes, there was no tumour. She had surgery immediately but that wasn't the problem. The prognosis for hypercalcaemia like this is very poor. I've known for some time I have to be prepared for that.'

They got into the lift together, in silence.

'Have you had any ideas about what might have caused it?'

'I really don't know. I did wonder if, maybe, it could have been her own mind.'

Michael looked forward, while his companion looked at him. 'My wife is a very creative woman and sometimes her imagination can run out of control.'

'You think it's a hysterical condition, then? I wonder if such a thing would be possible.'

'We can't rule it out, though it's a surprising idea, I know. But like a lot of artistic people, she has a very powerful irrationality, I suppose you could call it. Her creative mind can also be destructive in my experience of her. It could just as easily be a self-destructive force.'

'It sounds like it must have been very difficult.'

'Well, when all's said and done, she was, is, my wife. I have a duty to the children, as well as to her.'

'Have you considered vitamin D?'

Michael looked round to the man's face, without speaking, as the other became aware that they were uncomfortably close to each other.

'I mean – given your background, your interests.'

'What do you mean?' Michael said.

'Well, I assume you would have flagged up vitamin D overdose, if they hadn't already looked at it, as a trigger for hypercalcaemia?'

'I think that's rather farfetched.'

'Do you think so?'

The lift had stopped. Michael looked back at the doors, which were slow to open.

'I'm not sure how, or why, you think my wife overdosed on vitamins. Without my knowing, as her husband.'

'It's a well-known link though, isn't it? I say "well-known". For biological chemists like us it is, possibly not for a GP or a busy hospital doctor. It would take some time, of course. Hyper-dosing daily over a period of several weeks, I should think, before tipping over into an acute metabolic crisis.'

Michael walked out as the lift doors opened.

'I hope I haven't caused offence, it's just that vitamin D overdose is probably the working diagnosis, isn't it? Where there's no other explanation for a hypercalcaemic patient?'

He was talking to Michael's back, before he turned.

'I'm sure the hospital has assayed for excess vitamin D,' Michael said. 'If they had found it, they would have told me.'

'Well, you'd hope so. But it isn't that easy to do.' He was warming to the subject, unaware that Michael was not.

'I suppose she had only non-specific signs of poisoning by then. Vomiting, delirium, hallucinations, visions, flying sensations, that kind of thing. It just shows that anything can be potentially lethal in the right quantity. Or the wrong one. Who was it who said the poison is in the dose?'

'Paracelsus,' Michael said.

'It's interesting, isn't it?'

Michael didn't answer.

'Just to let you know,' the man began again. 'Between ourselves, I had a call about you. From somebody, well, high up. The reference he gave was very positive.'

'I'm glad,' Michael said.

'But I don't know what Analytical Labs really does. Analytical is only on our radar for animal feed. But I don't see you as an animal feed sort of a man. Is it classified?'

'Well, I could tell you,' Michael said, smiling. 'But then I'd have to kill you.'

31

Our mother's mysterious illness was just another fact of our childhood, which we both knew about but never questioned. Years later, after it was over, she sometimes suggested that Dad had poisoned her. But we never took her seriously, about that and many other things. There was no reason at the time to think she believed anything more sinister than that rejection and abandonment had been poison of a spiritual kind; that after my dad left, she'd experienced corrosive and highly toxic sadness.

But looked at with hindsight, the timing isn't consistent with my mother's illness being a somatised form of despair. She was suddenly and acutely ill long before she discovered that my dad no longer loved her, when she still thought he cared enough to keep her alive. Nobody will ever know the cause, at least for certain. It was several years before she was able to walk, and she remained fragile and easily tired. Calcium had worn away at her organs, like sand in an engine; she had several operations on her kidneys. The effect on her mind may also have been lasting.

My brother often says the past isn't real. Which is true, in many ways. For much of my working life, I've been a lawyer, which, without being in any way cynical, is all about storytelling and the past. In nearly every case, I took someone else's story and told it again, but with a different emphasis, one that placed them in a better light.

If a crime might have been committed a very long time ago, many would say too long ago to matter, then it's possible to speculate endlessly, to move the pieces this way and that way forever and reach a different conclusion every time.

Now I know that my dad was capable of fraud and subterfuge, and that he was unusually lacking in moral restraint, my mother's illness seems as suspicious as it was unexplained.

32

My brother has a case in the small claims court. He's irritated about not being paid some winnings by an online bookmaker. I've gone for a walk with him, hoping to persuade him to settle.

'It's not worth it,' I say. 'You can't get your costs back, so you'll spend much more in wasted time than you can recover.'

'It's the principle of the thing,' he says, smiling. 'But you're right. I'll drop it.'

'Good. Move on, it's for the best.'

'I've never really thought about it, but was it a coincidence, do you think?' my brother asks. 'That dad got into so much legal trouble and you became a lawyer?'

'It might have made me think about it,' I say. 'But I didn't go to Bar school until I was thirty. And before that, I had to go back and start again, to get the qualifications I needed to get in.'

'Neither of us was very stellar academically, at least the first time around. Maybe all that stuff about him sowed a seed in your mind. Because of where and how you last saw him, on his way to see a barrister and all that.'

I have considered this many times.

'I think he was probably right about me, in those days,' I say. 'What I was like up until he died. I was all over the place, to be honest.'

'If anything, I was doing even worse,' my brother says. 'I'd failed in my first attempt to get a maths degree and was working as a bookie's runner. Maybe we'd both missed out.'

'But, then again: so what? I really had no excuse for being like I was in my twenties. I had my own two feet to stand on, but I chose to make a mess of everything. And to keep on messing up.'

'It might have helped you, though. Helped both of us. If he'd been there.'

'I don't really believe in all that stuff,' I say. '"My dad was a this, so I was a that" sort of thing. Not either way round. It's reductive and it's just blame-shifting. I don't think anybody makes somebody else into the greatest success or the worst of failures. Sooner or later, we all have to own what we are and what we do.'

'That's probably how Dad thought about life too,' my brother says. 'Believing he could take on the whole world. And it was certainly how it ended, in a great big mess of his own making.'

'I'm not sure about what happened in the middle.'

'In the middle, was us,' my brother says.

'And those fake degrees.'

We walk on for a while in silence.

33

I saw Marie Lyon for the first time in the Sky TV documentary, *Primodos: A Bitter Pill*. She now leads a campaign group, the Association for Children Damaged by Hormone Pregnancy Tests, which was formed in 1978. Before Primodos took over her life, Marie would probably have called herself a mum from Wigan. Her daughter was born in 1970 without a left hand or the lower part of her left arm, after Marie had been given Primodos as a pregnancy test.

Energetic, business-like and single-minded, Marie looks much younger than she really is. But Primodos has cast a long shadow since she was given those two white pills when she was twenty-four years old and pregnant. I arranged to meet her because, strangely, we had something in common.

A group of legal claims were launched with the association's support against Bayer Schering in 1980, but they were stayed indefinitely in 1982 due to the lack of clear evidence that Primodos was to blame. As the case was being prepared for trial, a television programme called *The Primodos Affair* was made, but it was banned from being broadcast before it could be screened. Schering said the programme breached their right to confidentiality because the filmmakers had previously been given privileged access to Schering's inner workings and to its witnesses. The programme featured Schering's then witness, my dad. Marie has an idea what he said but, like everyone else, she is banned from watching the programme, even today.

Marie has believed for a very long time that my dad made decisions as a Schering scientist that resulted in her daughter being born without her lower left arm. If Isabel Gal had been listened to and believed, Marie Lyon would never have been given Primodos. It would have been taken off the market in 1967. So, somebody with my name – my surname – anyway – has been the enemy for several decades.

Marie hugged me before she spoke.

'What your dad did is absolutely not something you should ever feel responsible for,' she said.

I found out from her about what had happened in the court case, and that Marie never met my dad.

'I'm not sure whose witness he was in the end,' she said. 'Maybe he disappeared first from our side to join theirs. Then he wasn't there on their side either, at least by 1982. They seemed very reluctant to talk about why they dropped him. Whenever your dad's name came up, their lawyers seemed very nervous, they changed the subject. Our barrister thought they were hiding something about him but I've no idea what.'

'You do know about the scandal – in 1986, in the *Sunday Times*? About the fake research?'

'Oh yes,' Marie said. 'I even raised it with our legal team, back when you could've called it a team. They tried to argue that Schering's case was flawed because of your dad for that reason, but it didn't get anywhere. What he did in 1986 wasn't connected to Primodos.'

I told her about my dad's fake PhD degree and she laughed.

'Frankly, I'm not surprised', she said. 'But it's too late now in the court case to try to argue anything new. We have no choice – we have to go on what we've got. There's better expert evidence now. Professor Vargesson at Aberdeen University thinks he can finally prove what happened.'

In 2015, Marie Lyon had a stroke of luck. All the papers from the first Primodos court case were thought for many years to have been lost. But Marie discovered that they had all been copied and lodged in a Berlin library for safe keeping by a German prosecutor. No prosecution of Schering ever took place, but the papers remained and were disclosed. These old papers include confidential material from inside the Schering organisation. Together with new research demonstrating a link between foetal malformations in fish and Primodos-like hormones, this seemed to be the evidence they had been looking for.

'How's the case going now?'

'We've only got one lawyer left, who's doing the case for nothing,' she said. 'There's a mountain of paperwork, as you can imagine. And the government and Bayer Schering have applied to strike us out, so that really would be the end.'

Despite the newly discovered archive material and the recent scientific studies, clear proof still eluded them. Marie's organisation struggled to get legal representation this time round: they were just a group of ordinary families coping with extraordinary difficulties, they had little money and no Legal Aid anymore. Conditional fee solicitors came and went, then one or two pro bono barristers worked on the case when they could. When nobody else could do it, the task fell on Marie Lyon. She faced a tidal wave of technical material on top of the procedural demands of High Court litigation. Her small spare bedroom was packed full of documents about Primodos.

'The Cumberlege report has given us a little bit of hope again,' Marie said.

'The Cumberlege situation is complicated,' I said. 'Her conclusion is sympathetic but it wasn't in her remit to find fault, was it?'

'Schering and the government are having none of it, anyway. They don't have to beat us at all if this goes on long enough. They know the victims can't live forever. They're obviously a lot older now than they were the last time around, in 1982 – most in their sixties. They have complex health needs, congenital heart, lung and kidney problems. Sadly, we're losing people we love all the time.'

'But didn't Baroness Cumberlege recommend that they should all get compensation?' I said.

'There are no plans for a fund like thalidomide, if that's what you mean. Or anything like it. With Primodos, despite what Baroness Cumberlege said, it's still like it all never happened. So, we are pinning our hopes on the court case, for the time being.'

I could have told Marie a lot more about my dad's fraudulent life, about the complicated story of the blue book and the red book together, but I didn't. I wanted to, but it sounded irrelevant and farfetched when I started saying it out loud. Marie's case was facing an extinction event after over three decades of effort. Telling her tales about a scientist who wasn't there risked making a bad situation worse, by distracting her from the final battle or offering false hope of a solution.

34

'The thing is, if I don't tell her everything I know and the Primodos victims get nothing – do you think that makes me a bit responsible too?'

I've gone to see my brother, trying to work out how I feel after talking to Marie Lyon. I've been exposed to a stranger's involvement in a situation we've treated up to now as purely a family affair.

'No, not at all,' he says. 'And she said the same. It's much too late in the case and of questionable relevance. The thalidomide compensation didn't rely on some charlatan being responsible for causing it.'

'Though there was never a court judgment about thalidomide,' I say. 'The case was settled, and for much less than what they asked for. Thalidomide is still called a "tragic event" that nobody could have foreseen.'

Thalidomide was withdrawn in the UK in 1961, within weeks of a letter in the *Lancet*. Australian obstetrician William McBride reported a sudden increase in the number of babies with birth defects being born at a women's hospital in Sydney. His letter was only five sentences long and invited other clinicians to share their experiences. The manufacturer, Distillers, wrote to the *Lancet* in December 1961 announcing that it was withdrawing the drug. It was never licensed again for pregnant women, although it is an effective treatment for some malignant cancers.

By contrast, after Isabel Gal's letter was published in 1967, nothing really happened at all. Three years' later, Primodos was labelled as a treatment for irregular periods, but the new warning about giving it to pregnant women wasn't widely publicised. The persistence of the 'toad is slow' advertising slogan and wrongly labelled sample packets still hanging around in surgeries probably led to several further years of mis-prescribing, until Primodos was withdrawn altogether in 1978.

In his autobiography, the UK health regulator William Inman – that man who had been in touch with my dad and later admitted destroying files of data about Primodos – said the lesson from the 'unpredictable tragedy' of thalidomide was that 'no manufacturer could be relied on to monitor or make "sell-or-withdraw" decisions on his product'. But Inman's failure to intervene with Schering indicates that he believed the opposite. The thalidomide tragedy gave Inman the idea to write to the Department of Health and offer to have himself appointed as the nation's gatekeeper for drug safety. He was also an expert witness in the 1980s in a case in the USA about a hormone pregnancy test said to have caused foetal harm, giving evidence on the side of the drug's manufacturer.

'The Primodos claim has been listed for another hearing,' I tell my brother. 'Back again, like Jarndyce and Jarndyce.'

'Like what?'

'Like the never-ending case in Dickens' *Bleak House*. I can understand the legal side of it, if not the science. It's been inactive since 1982, so most of the witnesses are dead. Marie Lyon asked me if I wanted to go along and listen.'

'And will you?' my brother asks.

'I promised Marie I would. It's not a hearing of evidence, it's a strike-out. If the other side succeeds, the case will be killed off for good.'

35

After our meeting, Marie sent me some letters sent between my dad and a mathematician in 1967 and 1968, about neonatal deformity statistics. I ran my finger over his signature, which is in some ways more familiar to me than his face. He used to write postcards, which stood in for him in his absence. I could never throw the letters away, although I don't know where they went.

I printed them out and took them to my brother's.

❊ ❊ ❊

'This first one is to a statistician, Dennis Cook,' I say. 'In a previous letter, which I haven't got, Cook must have suggested setting up a big Primodos safety trial. Dad says he can't. He rubbishes Isabel Gal's research methods, but then he says:

> "*The apparent correlation between the increase in congenital malformations and the sale of pregnancy diagnosis pills <u>looks rather alarming</u>. I appreciate that correlations can be misleading, but we are here <u>dealing with a pharmaceutical product taken by pregnant women that may be capable of altering the chemical environment of the foetus</u> and I think we will have to be ultra-cautious in this matter.*"

'In other words: Dad understood the risk.'

'But a coincidence of two things doesn't prove that one caused the other,' my brother says. 'Correlation can be a strong indication of causation, but it's not the same.'

'You need to see the reasons why he is ruling out a further study,' I say, handing him the letter. 'He says it would be a "large undertaking". But what is "large" for an international pharmaceutical company? If they wanted to do it, they could just do it. He obviously knows the real problem is that, and I quote: ". . . it would draw widespread attention to the suggested side-effect of the tablets, and this in itself would probably prevent the completion of such a trial".'

'In other words,' my brother says, 'if pregnant women recruited to a study found out what it was all about, then they wouldn't take the pills.'

'"Suggested side-effect" is quite an understatement, isn't it? But moving on to Cook's response. He now has even more to say about correlation because he's received the rest of the data. He's got national figures for Primodos distribution and the incidence of birth defects from 1959. He's drawn a graph and he says: "There is a strong correlation, with a coefficient of 0.78."'

'That's a strong positive correlation between the drug and birth defects,' says my brother. 'The scale is from zero, no correlation, to one, perfect positive correlation.'

'Cook concludes that "the present evidence is strong enough to demand a serious follow-up to Dr Gal's findings". But is high correlation the same as scientific proof?'

'Some people will never be satisfied. They will still want to put their fist in the wound.'

We look at the letters for a while without speaking. I'm looking at my dad's familiar, looping handwriting in blue ink, from his fountain pen.

'Who looked after us most of the time, when we were small?' I ask my brother.

'That I don't know,' my brother says. 'It's another mystery.'

☆ ☆ ☆

To get another perspective, I see a friend who's likely to have an opinion. She's a research psychologist and she knows a lot about quantitative research methods.

As we make lunch, I tell her about the conversation with my brother.

'Well, all research has got its strengths and its weaknesses,' she says. 'If you look at the Gal study in 1967, there's obviously a potential problem with this stuff and birth defects. In the letter, your dad criticises Dr Gal for not matching the cases and controls geographically. But I'd call what she's done a pretty good case-control study. There's nothing wrong with it. She's studying something that's already happened, so she's comparing the affected group with some similar unaffected people to see if there's a causal factor that jumps out.'

'What could Isabel Gal have done instead?' I ask her.

'I don't think she had many other choices,' she says. 'Maybe she could have matched for other factors. Socio-economic status is big in pregnancy outcomes, so is smoking. It's an imperfect case-control study but it's good enough. The gold standard would be a randomised controlled trial, of course. Expensive, difficult. And, more to the point, unethical.'

'Isn't that what my dad is saying in the letter?'

'Well, yeah,' she says, 'in a way. But after the statistical analysis, not before. By then, he knows the risks are obviously too high, so he can't do a proper randomised study. No sane woman would volunteer for a study like that.'

'Absence of evidence isn't evidence of absence, of course,' I say.

'But you might pretend it is, if you're scared to look too closely. These days, the ethics committee would stop what Cook is suggesting in its tracks. But the 1968 letters suggest they were planning a Primodos study with a group of 200 GPs. Which sounds mad! Then this drug stays on the market for years and years anyway. It makes no sense to me.'

'Tell me what you think about the statistics,' I say.

'Well, Cook has made a logarithmic graph but it's got lost. It was based on birth defect figures compared with the distribution of Primodos throughout the country from 1957 to 1961. He says he thinks there's a strong correlation and I do too. A coefficient of 0.78 is a very high number in social science research. But also interesting: he sees "high initial scatter".'

'What does that mean?' I say.

'If you can picture this graph, it has, say, birth defect numbers along the bottom axis and Primodos supply figures up the side. "Scatter" means dots all over the place, so the two things you're measuring are less connected. As the coefficient gets higher, the relationship comes together as more of a line until at coefficient 1.0, you get a straight diagonal line. Perfect correlation. By 1961, this coefficient 0.78 would be dots clustering closely around the diagonal, whereas previously it was less clear.'

'Why might that have been?'

'Well, presumably something has started happening in about 1961 that made Primodos more closely correlated with birth defects than it was before. Or something *stopped* happening that was creating "noise" behind the Primodos-to-birth-defect coefficient. It would have to be some other cause for the same kind of birth defects.'

'There was thalidomide, of course. Marketed in the UK from 1958 and withdrawn in 1961.'

'Maybe,' she says. 'Thalidomide also affected pregnant women, not the same numbers or distribution, but it also caused birth defects. So, it's plausible. And, to be honest, what else could it possibly be, affecting the whole country? A cloud of space dust?'

36

May 2023, Royal Courts of Justice, Strand, London

Wilson and others v. Bayer Pharma

In Charles Dickens' fictional court case of Jarndyce v. Jarndyce, a judge stares into a lantern with no light in it, surveying a sea of wigs, stuck in a fogbank. Fortunately, the legal system has moved on since then.

When I was a barrister, the Royal Courts of Justice was a place of work. But in the spring of 2023, I went there for the first time as a spectator. Bayer Schering and the government had applied to strike out the Primodos claim, ensuring it could never come back to court. Marie Lyon had managed to scrape together a legal team to face the onslaught.

I hadn't been for a while, but the huge vaulted and tiled main hall still felt familiar to me. The air inside was cool and damp, like a cathedral. The main hall sits in the middle of a tangled skein of corridors, twisting and turning, up and down stone staircases, each thread leading eventually to one of over a hundred courtrooms. Some are vast and grand, lined to the rooflights with red-bound and blue-bound books. Others are very small, scarcely more than cupboards. In the basement, the light and the ceilings are low, and the floors are grey concrete rather than coloured mosaic tile. Some of these courts have heavy wooden lancet doors with cast iron latches, like a fairy door among the roots of an old tree.

The Primodos claim was last looked at in this building in 1982. Back then, the judge had put the case into a deep procedural sleep, so that the plaintiffs, as they were called in the legal language of those days, could try to get better expert evidence. Future scientific advances might help explain the cause of their disabilities, whether Primodos was likely to have been to blame, and if so, precisely how.

When I found the daily Cause List posted in the main hall in the Strand, I discovered that the hearing wasn't happening in this building at all. It was scheduled in a room at the new Rolls Building, five minutes' walk away, in Fetter Lane.

The Rolls Building was opened only a decade ago, and its court rooms are designed for twenty-first-century litigation. When Victorian architects designed court buildings, they were thinking in portrait, visualising cases with two sides, with judgment being handed down from a high dais in the middle. They were building churches of the law, with aisles and pews, and an ecclesiastical idea of where justice might come from.

The Rolls Building has landscape courtrooms, for modern, multi-party proceedings. These are secular, wide-open spaces, more like a conference centre than a church.

The judge in this new Primodos case was a thirteen-year-old schoolgirl when the previous version came to a temporary end. Court bundles are now electronic and accessed through monitors. There aren't any wigs and gowns anymore either, but you can still tell who would have been wearing them. They're at the front, comfortable in this strange environment, sitting on the desks before the judge arrives or mingling like the hosts at a party. There are invisible lines running crossways through the room. They divide the claimants from the respondents, and all the lawyers together away from everyone else.

I joined a group of people dressed in street clothes, in what is still called a public gallery. It's no longer a high vantage point but a row of chairs at the back of the courtroom, where those claimants who were physically able had gathered with their families to watch their own case as spectators. We were cut off from the proceedings and could barely hear what was being said. We watched the scene together, like theatregoers with an obstructed view at the very back of the stalls.

The respondents' three King's Counsel attacked the claimants' case one after the other, in a coordinated and sustained assault over many hours. They said that the claimants failed to be specific enough in the pleadings about who it was that suffered which sort of malformation. They said their genetic tests were irrelevant – and even if they weren't, they didn't exclude natural causes for all their many problems. The claimants had asked all the wrong questions of the wrong kind of experts, who had considered all the wrong things. Expert groups had exonerated Primodos long ago, particularly the Expert Working Group in 2017, and in this, the judge had no choice but to follow suit. Expensive legal minds professed themselves baffled: it all happened too long ago they said, with a sorrowful shrug. And if that wasn't enough, the claimants had no idea how the claim would be paid for. So, it had to fail.

I knew very well why these things were being said, as a lawyer. As a human being, I think it could have been said with more respect for people who have faced undeniable difficulties, whatever the cause. I now understood, from sitting in a public gallery, why the courts made so little sense to the Primodos claimants. For them, the whole thing lacked any common sense or decency. There were simple questions, as they saw it, that nobody on the other side had ever answered.

Like: If your daughter or your sister were pregnant, would you give her Primodos?

Or: If you were pregnant, would you take it yourself?

Or: If Primodos was perfectly safe, then why was it withdrawn?

Or: How did a pregnancy test come to be labelled, as it was in 1970, 'unsafe for pregnant women'?

Unfortunately, from the claimants' point of view, the questions needing answers had become stuck in the fogbank.

❉ ❉ ❉

As I left the courtroom, a woman touched my elbow and then took hold of my hands.

'I knew your father,' she said, 'and I spoke to your mother. The day after your father left you all. She was so distressed and crying. She was in hell.'

Sandy Malcolm had been the receptionist at Schering's head office in Burgess Hill from 1967 until 1971, when she went on maternity leave. When Sandy thought she might be pregnant, she went upstairs to the executive floor and asked if she could have Primodos, so she could find out for certain. A senior scientist refused to give it to her.

'He told me it might cause birth defects, so I shouldn't take it. I suppose he didn't want what happened to all these people to happen to me.'

I asked her if she remembered anything else about my dad.

'We didn't know they'd been having an affair until the two of them suddenly left. That was in 1970. They both disappeared and then we heard they'd settled in Africa.'

'Yes, in Zambia,' I said.

'One of their secretaries stayed in touch. She was told they lost a baby. Late on, at seven months.'

'Yeah, I heard that too,' I said.

37

'They've lost. The Primodos claim has been struck out.'

It's June 2023, and the judgment has just been published.

'Oh dear, that's disappointing for them,' my brother says. 'Though not really unexpected, was it?'

'They couldn't pay lawyers, so their barristers and expert witnesses were doing the case for free. The fact that they couldn't afford to run the case was a factor, which seems so unfair. They had Legal Aid last time, in 1982. But the world has changed.'

'Apart from lack of money, what else?'

'The science hasn't changed enough to prove that Primodos caused their disabilities. There's a suggested mechanism, that the drug temporarily cuts off the oxygen supply to the foetus. But the scientists can't agree. Then there's the statistics. But the statistics hardly featured, for some reason.'

'Speaking as a mathematician, lawyers and statistics aren't a happy combination,' my brother says.

'It's always been a problem for the claimants that there have been previous investigations that didn't support what they were saying. Particularly the Expert Working Group, the EWG. The EWG said in 2017 there was no causal link. The judge relied on the EWG, among other things. So maybe the writing has been on the wall for the victims' group since then.'

'I suppose they'll never get – what do they call it these days? Closure?' my brother says.

'Probably not. But the judge did say one surprising thing. She said if it could be proved that the case in 1982 had been "infected by improper conduct", then that might have been a reason for the claim to carry on.'

'Who could she be thinking of, I wonder?' my brother says.

'Well, she must have meant Dad. And the 1986 scandal, I suppose.'

'Did you tell Marie Lyon about that?'

'I didn't need to. She already knew about the *Sunday Times* thing. Everybody does. Her lawyers said a while ago that it wasn't relevant because there was no nexus with the Primodos timing, the 1960s. But the point now is that if Dad wasn't ever qualified to manage Primodos safely or to do the necessary research, then maybe the blue and red books really are the missing link.'

38

Earlier in these proceedings, it was suggested that the previous litigation may have been infected by improper conduct on the part of experts connected to the defendants whose research has since been called into question. That is something that would not have been in the contemplation of the parties or Bingham J in 1982 but which might, if substantiated, amount to a good reason to allow the matter to be reopened. However, that aspect was not pursued and I have seen no evidence that any impropriety affected the outcome of [the] previous claim.

Mrs Justice Yip,
The Primodos strike-out decision, Wilson and
others v. Bayer Pharma AG and others, 2023

Nobody could have known in 1982 – not the judge, nor the plaintiffs, or probably even Schering – that my dad would soon be caught up in a scientific scandal. The investigation of his conduct at Deakin was about to begin as that court case was ending, and what he'd done would not become public knowledge for another four years.

But this more recent version of the case, in 2023, started over thirty years after the scandal. Nothing said in the *Sunday Times* in 'The Bogus Work of Professor Briggs' has ever been contradicted. Was it the 1986 research scandal that Mrs Justice Yip was talking about?

If so, it seemed that the claimants had stopped trying to rely on it. A small, pro-bono legal team had to train its limited ammunition on a small number of targets, and time was short. The possibility that the earlier 1980 proceedings had been tainted because my dad would, within a few years, be brought down by a scandal, did not gain any traction. My dad's conduct in 1986 seemed too remote from decisions he made about Primodos in 1966–70 to be considered relevant. An argument like this might even have had a whiff of desperation about it. Just because he was involved in a scandal, that wouldn't necessarily negate his entire career.

But what if everything he ever did was founded on deliberate pretence?

Over the next few months, I thought a lot about the Primodos judgment. At the same time, Marie Lyon and the other Primodos claimants were being pursued for court costs by both Bayer Schering and the UK government. A group of sick and disabled people were being asked to pay over a million pounds or, presumably, be bankrupted.

Something else was also bothering me. Even though I'd stopped 'all that ferreting around', as my brother had started to call it, I had the uncomfortable feeling that my dad's fabrications, both big and small, would have more serious and far-reaching consequences than I'd previously realised.

Whether my dad's opinions were valid about meteorites, or even about the whole of Mars, it was unlikely to matter very much.

In the field of human hormones, however, my dad's questionable research could have become so tightly woven into the fabric of scientific understanding that the fact and the fake may be indistinguishable from each other.

If this was what had happened, then thankfully it is extremely unlikely to be putting the users of oral contraceptives at risk today. My dad's fraudulent research was uncovered in 1986; since then, there have been hundreds of further studies, each one adding a further well-founded layer to the sum of understanding. But the same can't be said about Primodos, a substance that belongs to the past. There is no more research being done by the companies that used to make hormone pregnancy tests. All that remains is historic, mainly the archived, in-house studies. The few researchers today who are trying to recreate the conditions for alleged Primodos harm, in university departments and with comparatively little funding, can only ethically study the effects of similar chemicals on zebra fish. Some scientists now believe that a hormone spike from Primodos tablets could cause contractions like early labour, disrupt tiny blood vessels in the developing limbs and organs of the foetus, or bring on a miscarriage. But it remains a hypothesis that decision-makers are reluctant to accept because the old material does not seem to support it.

Evidence of my dad's reckless personality long before the 1980s research fraud, in the invention of his doctoral degree, had a bearing on the Primodos story after all. Once I knew he didn't have a doctorate, and that he did little or nothing to get a DSc, and that he tended to write whatever he felt like writing then publish it, with little interest in scientific rigour, that raised the possibility that a closed subject like Primodos could still be actively infected with his ill-considered opinions.

The tide seemed to have turned against the Primodos claimants after the Expert Working Group decided that there was no
causal link to explain the pre-birth injuries and miscarriages. But
if the EWG had seen research papers produced my dad, without
any reason to know what kind of person he was, or that there was
any reason to doubt what he might say, and if they relied on that
research, then the group's findings would arguably be flawed.

The EWG closed down its investigation and disbanded in
2017. But the research studies and papers on which they based
their conclusions are still available online.

39

There's an electronic file called 'Schering Studies' with the Expert Working Group report on the government website. This is all the redacted documents which were not properly disclosed at Schering's request.

There are eighty-two papers inside, all of which have had the names of the authors, recipients and even locations obliterated with black marker. Most of them have dates, but how accurate the dates are is difficult to know because some are also marked 'in contemplation of litigation': in other words, they were created by Bayer Schering because the company was already being sued over Primodos. These documents look like reproductions of multiple earlier papers, which have been collected into anthologies so they can be presented more easily to a court and a judge.

There are four Primodos research papers in the 'Schering Studies' file from the period when my dad was UK research director between 1966 and 1970: three studies from 1970, one using rabbits as research subjects, and two with rats; and a study from 1968, with mice. This last paper is so characteristically in my dad's writing style, I could almost hear him reading it. It's a preliminary study, identifying the sample dose for a longer experiment with the main component of Primodos. The final report, dated 16 May 1968, was produced by someone whose name has been blocked out, who was based at my dad's office, the Schering building in Burgess Hill. I know it's him.

There's some beagle research in the Schering Studies, too. Both beagle study papers rely on past research done in my dad's name. I knew that my dad produced at least one reliable paper on beagles in collaboration with someone else, and maybe this beagle research was also carried out with an expert who knew what they were talking about. Or maybe not.

There is no doubt that the EWG considered research carried out by my dad, as well as other studies that were dependent on what he'd previously said, and still more whose unknown author could have been him. One of these papers is a follow-up study, intended to investigate a previous finding that foetal malformations had been caused by Primodos-like chemicals. But this second paper found, for reasons that are not clear from the paper itself, that there were no malformations at all. Nobody really knows how much influence these old experiments had on the ERG's conclusion that Primodos had no causal connection with the undeveloped limbs and digits, the misshapen and missing organs, and the miscarriages that seemed to follow its use.

Human research that could prove to everybody's satisfaction that Primodos caused birth defects would be unconscionable – a paradoxical situation in which Primodos is so potentially dangerous it can only be presumed to be safe.

40

In July 2015, I stood in this House and urged the Government to disclose all the evidence they had and to set up an independent inquiry. The then Minister, the hon. Member for Mid Norfolk (George Freeman), heard those concerns and agreed to an independent review, which would be led by an expert working group.

However, first, the expert working group was not independent. In fact, many of the experts were found to have conflicts of interest with the industry. Secondly, the review of the evidence conveniently ignored several important studies and then later said, 'Oh, well, there was insufficient evidence.' Thirdly, the terms of reference of the review had said that it would try to find a possible link. Yet the reports' conclusion said it was unable to find a 'causal link'. How exactly does the Government intend to find a causal link, short of testing the drug on pregnant women? . . .

I am pleased to see the right hon. Member for Maidenhead [Theresa May] in the Chamber. I know that, as Prime Minister at the time, she read this report. I note that in a recent Sky News interview she said:

'I felt that it wasn't the slam dunk answer that people said it was.'

Knowing what we now know, that the expert working group report was a whitewash, riddled with factual inaccuracies and conflicts of interest; knowing that studies from Oxford University

have proven that the evidence in this report was deliberately manip-
ulated to reach its conclusion; knowing that the Prime Minister
of the day knew something was not right and then commissioned
another review – how can it be right that any Government can
continue to use this report to hide their sins?

Only a few weeks ago, lawyers used the report in court to
defend their preposterous claims, and Ministers have used it as a
basis to refuse and deny families redress. It is outrageous. I ask
the Minister today: will she take a stand and do the right thing?
Will she be courageous and read beyond the lines of the ministe-
rial briefing she has been given? Only then will she agree with me
that the expert working group report is not worth the paper it is
written on.

Yasmin Qureshi MP
Hansard, 7 September 2023

The other thing that the Government have done is hide behind
the expert working group report, which the hon. Lady referred
to. Many issues have been related to the expert working group
report, which of course found in its overall conclusion that:

> '. . . the available scientific evidence, taking all aspects
> into consideration, does not support a causal association
> between the use of HPTs, such as Primodos, during early
> pregnancy and adverse outcomes, either with regard to
> miscarriage, stillbirth or congenital anomalies.'

Given that conclusion, it might seem rather strange to the Minister
and the House that it was that very report that led to my setting

up the Cumberlege review. The reason I did so was that earlier in the report it says:

> 'The totality of the available evidence from pharmacology, non-clinical, epidemiological and adverse event reporting data was very limited and did not, on balance, support a causal association between the use of HPTs, such as Primodos, by the mother during early pregnancy and congenital anomalies in the child.'

To me, 'on balance' means that there was an argument against a causal link and, on the other side, an argument for a causal link, so the strength of the absolute decision that the expert working group came out with was, I think, a misrepresentation of what they had put earlier in the report. It was that sense of a balanced argument that led me to call for the Cumberlege review.

Theresa May MP
former Prime Minister, 7 September 2023

41

'It's as if I can see Dad, you know. Through all the cracks in the Primodos case.'

'I think I know what you mean.'

'He was there at the scene, in the 1960s. At the very least, he shared responsibility for what happened, whatever it was. He probably said a lot of things in those nine minutes in *The Primodos Affair*. We will probably never know exactly what. But from what Yasmin Qureshi has seen and read into *Hansard*, he seems to have said that Primodos wouldn't have been licensed if had just been invented. After 1970, even the EWG thought that Schering did too little by today's standards to stop Primodos from being used as a pregnancy test. After they knew it shouldn't be.'

'He'd gone by then, of course. To Zambia.'

'Yes, true. He'd been having an affair in his office, we'll never know for how long. So work was to him an exciting place to be, full of romantic opportunities.'

'No wonder he was never at home. Apart from when he was trying to bump off our mum of course, according to you,' my brother says.

'How do you feel about that?' I ask him. 'It's quite possible he did try to poison her, it's a reasonable hypothesis. Though we'll never really know.'

'I know it sounds weird, but it doesn't really change how I feel about either of them. We weren't very kind to Mum sometimes, because she was a bit bonkers. Maybe that was why she was that way. But it doesn't make much difference to me.'

'What about him? I mean, seriously, trying to kill somebody?'

'Well, if he did – and it remains a big "if" – if he did, he was what he was, wasn't he? I feel like that sort of behaviour was baked-in to the price, as it were.'

'Marie Lyon and all the other women like her have been left with a lifetime of guilt. As mothers, they all feel they're to blame for what happened to their babies.

'Because no matter what they know logically, deep down they believe they should never have taken it. GPs with a load of old samples still in a drawer, dishing out tablets with no warnings on them.'

'The "Toad is Slow" was still in their minds, probably. It was a very memorable image. Very persuasive.'

'So, those GPs were probably trying to do their best as well. They were all let down, weren't they? In different ways,' I add.

'I don't think Dad had much experience of guilt,' my brother says. 'He'd have thought it was for little people.'

42

I have given my commitment from the Dispatch Box to review the outstanding recommendations in relation to Primodos, because I want to get to the bottom of this once and for all and provide justice for the families. I have heard from Members across the House about their concerns and the outstanding recommendations of the Cumberlege review, and my commitment is to look at those now.

Maria Caulfield MP, health minister
7 September 2023

In the House of Commons debate on 7 September 2023, despite the end of the court case and all the reviews and inquiries, there was still no answer to the problem of Primodos.

During the debate, many MPs talked about the experiences of constituents who had taken the drug, and the lives of their children. Dame Angela Eagle raised the case of Marjorie, whose daughter Tania has had complex heart and intestinal illness since birth, requiring frequent surgery. Suzanne Webb talked about Helen, whose daughter Beccy has severe developmental delay and has never walked. Ed Davey's constituent, Sue, died earlier in the year. Her daughter was born with multiple deformities and she has never lived independently. Jeff Smith had met Patricia, whose son was born without an arm. Patricia died in 2017, around the time that the EWG rebutted their claims as 'not causally linked' to Primodos. Edward and Janet's daughter Louise, now fifty-four, was born with multiple disabilities, including learning impairment, hearing loss and difficulty walking. Janet suffered a breakdown due to the strain of caring for her daughter. Without some kind of additional help, they do not know what will happen to Louise when they are no longer there to look after her.

It's impossible to know how culpable my dad really was in the Primodos story and whether what he did caused harm to the individuals and families who believe they are Primodos victims. Surely for their sake, the next inquiry, if there is one, must be the last.

My dad comes and goes as a character in the Primodos affair, and it's hard to pin down what he did or didn't do. It is worth remembering that, before the job at Schering, he had dealt only in abstract concepts, like space exploration and laboratory research. I'm not sure he ever understood his actions to have consequences for real people, like Tania, or Beccy, or Louise.

There are three distinct points of contact between my dad and the Primodos story, and I think the last is probably the most significant. When he met Isabel Gal in 1967, he was new to his job at Schering and, at thirty-one years of age, relatively young. From what we can see in his letters to the statistician Dennis Cook, he seemed to be enjoying the intellectual challenge of real-life science. These letters suggest he was genuinely trying to find an answer and that he was aware of the risks that synthetic hormones could pose in the environment of a growing foetus. But he had the power to do more than that.

Fast-forward nearly fifteen years to the months before the collapse of the first court case in 1982 and he appears to have wanted to express an opinion about Primodos on the victims' side, but something stopped him. Perhaps he drew back because he sensed that his reputation could be harmed. Maybe that's when he remembered that his CV was a fabrication and he foresaw being pulled apart in the witness box. He was older by then, in his late forties, with much more to lose in terms of money and professional standing, and nothing to gain by taking a risk like that.

Since his death, Schering has dug out of its archives some of the papers he wrote in the 1960s, to shore up their position in the Primodos argument. From the time when he wrote them until September 1986 at the latest, Schering could reasonably have claimed that this was the work of a responsible and conscientious expert in the field of synthetic hormone research. After 1986, that confidence had to be misplaced. Perhaps the company was still reassured by the fact that, whatever frauds he might have committed, he was still a top-flight scientist with a string of publications and two doctoral degrees to his name.

One or two of my dad's books can still be found in second-hand warehouses. Nothing he wrote alone should ever be relied on, though it seems, perhaps, that the Expert Working Group did. My dad's fake qualifications are now in the mix as well, adding yet another layer of concern about the material on which the EWG based its conclusions. After the 1986 research scandal, everything my dad had ever written or published was judged likely to be worthless, and none of it is there anymore, in the libraries and specialist collections where it used to be.

From what I can remember, my dad's own bookshelves had surprisingly few scientific texts on them, apart from the not insignificant number he'd written himself. *Fantastic Stories* and *Astounding* magazines were lovingly preserved in matching binders, and the rest were mainly paperbacks. He liked comic books, with strip cartoons in them rather than text. When he closed the door of his study to spend time alone, he would lose himself again in the space-age comics of his childhood. Then he might pick up a novel with a bright cover, showing a burnt orange desert on Jupiter, a cosmonaut escaping a solar flare or a silver disc flying over a Martian city, and he would drift into an imaginary future with Ray Bradbury, Isaac Asimov and Arthur C Clarke.

PART 3

SCIENCE FICTION

'So much has been done, exclaimed the soul of Frankenstein – more, far more, will I achieve . . .'

Victor Frankenstein
Frankenstein by Mary Shelley

43

Michael pushed his way through the crowd on the pavement outside the cinema, reaching behind him to catch hold of Marion's hand. Once they were again side by side, he interlaced his fingers with hers, inside the pocket of his overcoat.

'So – what did you think of it? The film.'

'I thought it was very romantic,' she said.

'Romantic? Really? In what way?'

'I suppose because of how much she, Louise that is, really loves Scott. She really, truly loves him, even in spite of everything that happens. She wants to stay married to him no matter what. Even when his hand is too small to keep his wedding ring from falling off.'

She pressed her thumb momentarily into the crease where his ring finger met his palm.

'Even when he's so small he has to live in the doll's house. When there's no hope of them ever having a normal life again, she still wants them to be together. I think that's really romantic. And sad, too, of course.'

'Oh, don't be daft!' he said, laughing. 'It's science fiction. It's not supposed to be romantic.'

'I know that. But you asked me what I felt. And I can't help how I feel.'

Michael made a wide, frustrated gesture with his free arm, while his other hand responded to her touch, gently holding her thumb.

'Look,' he said, catching her eye for a second. 'Think about the scene when they're on the boat. Louise goes below the deck to get him a beer and while she's gone, the phosphorescent cloud covers him with drops. It's a random event, it's completely random that it's him and not her. But it changes Scott's chemistry. And as he shrinks, he adapts. D'you see? What it's saying is, there is no Fate. There's no point in having supernatural beliefs or superstitions. There's only chance and a man's will to win. Life is an arbitrary test of character, pure and simple. It's a trial of what makes us human.'

'I do see what you mean,' Marion said. 'But I still believe there are mysteries. There are hidden patterns everywhere. It's not easy to see the future but not because it isn't there. I think so, anyway.'

They began to walk more slowly, separated from their surroundings by a new silence.

'Sometimes I think I recognise you,' he said. 'Like all of this has happened before.'

She smiled and looked away.

'Anyway,' he said, 'isn't it a bit cruel to pretend to Scott that everything's all right? To lie to him?'

'I don't think she's lying to him, at all. She's not stupid, Michael. Louise can see he's changed, that he's still changing, but he's still Scott. So, she loves him.'

'Even when he's so small he's battling spiders with a darning needle?'

'You're making fun of me now.'

'No, I'm not, I'm serious – even when he's a speck of dust, an atomic particle? Will Louise still love him then?'

'I believe so. That's what love is.'

Michael laughed and pulled her tightly into his side.

'Love is just chemicals, Marion. It's not magic, it's just simple chemical reactions, that's all. Just biology and chemistry working together. We are all just big sacks of chemical soup, when it comes to it.'

'You don't really believe that – do you?' Marion stopped to look up into his eyes. 'I don't think you do. Not really. And Scott believes that God can see him too. No matter how small he is. God sees him.'

'We are all of us infinitesimally small in the universe,' Michael replied. 'That's all there is to it, I'm afraid. Even so-called God.'

44

My mother never said exactly when it was that she met my dad, although I never noticed this omission at the time. But now, when I look back down the years at them, as if through a hag stone, there were signs in the way their relationship began that revealed its frangible essence and foreshadowed its end.

In the spring of 1957, my dad was about to lose the next two years of his life to National Service, unless he could get out of the country before September. But escape would require a whole new start somewhere else. His science degree and teaching diploma would get him a job somewhere, in a school probably, but he already knew he would never be content with that.

In his first twenty years, he'd travelled less than fifty miles. He'd left his parents' home in Chadderton, a mill town on the road from Manchester to Oldham, for university in Liverpool. In the mid-1950s, Liverpool was a city entering a period of post-industrial decline and had yet to begin recovering from Blitz bombing.

My dad was the only child of older parents. His father, Harry, had grown up in Hulme, an area of inner-city slums and deprivation at the time, so he was never destined to achieve his dream of becoming an engineer. He was a typewriter repair man, a taciturn presence in their small house and full of bottled-up resentment. My dad's mother, Flo, was probably lonely, so she channelled all her hopes into her only son, doting on him. By the time he turned eighteen, my dad was keen to escape. When my dad finished his chemistry degree, he'd stayed on for a year to get a teaching certificate, moving from a student bedsit to a rented room in a run-down house near Garston match works. He walked to the university library every day along grimy streets pock-marked with derelict buildings. Toxic smog filled his lungs and stung his eyes. The long, wet winters were worse than the disappointingly cool summers, without very much to choose between them.

My dad knew by then that his character would not be suited to a small life. To an ordinary, disappointed life, like his father's. But given where he was, and what he was, there was no bigger life available to be had.

Although Liverpool still had one advantage left for him. When he knew what to do, he could escape it with ease, by sea.

❖ ❖ ❖

In May 1957, my mother turned twenty-one. She was small and slight, barely five feet and one inch tall, and, in the language of the time, she was elfin in appearance. She always wore her dark hair cropped very short to her head in a modern, boyish style and she had an art student's elan, even though she'd left school at fifteen to work as a seamstress. At the time, Marion usually dressed in the beatnik uniform of calf-length pencil skirt, ballet pumps and beret, though she was neither radical nor intellectual. She had instead a kind of aesthetic intuition, and a sense of everyday magic all around her.

Having both arrived at a university ball with other people, Michael and Marion danced together without really speaking, then were curiously reluctant to part at the end of the night. The following day, my dad hung around outside the dress factory where my mother was working and persuaded her to go with him to the cinema. They went to see the new release, *The Incredible Shrinking Man*, a film about an apparently insignificant event with life-changing consequences.

A few days after their first date, my dad was offered a job at a further education college in Montreal, based on a letter he'd sent over six months before. He'd never believed in luck and yet now his fortunes had mysteriously started to improve. Perhaps Marion was a talisman. Maybe only she needed to believe in magic for them both to benefit.

On 24 July 1957, the day after Michael's last exam, my parents left Liverpool docks for Canada on the SS *Carinthia*.

This transatlantic sailing is the second of the two immoveable events that marked the beginning and end of this chapter in my parents' relationship, when they turned from strangers into a husband and a wife. *The Incredible Shrinking Man* had to be on in cinemas when it began. And they had to be on board the SS *Carinthia* when it left Liverpool docks on that particular Wednesday, in time for the happy ending. Happy, at least, for the time being.

The Incredible Shrinking Man premiered in Manhattan in February 1957 and was not showing in local cinemas in America or worldwide until at least two months later. So, it couldn't have been on at the Futurist in Lime Street, Liverpool, before April or possibly even May of that year. My parents can only have known each other for a matter of weeks, certainly less than three months, when they left the country together on one-way tickets to Canada.

My dad had his twenty-second birthday in Montreal, as a married man. They'd had a quick civil ceremony on arrival, without any guests and with town hall staff as witnesses.

It's hard to imagine my parents as I knew them being caught up in a whirlwind romance. But if it was called rashness or impulsivity, then that would be much easier to believe about them both. Neither of my parents was by nature either cautious or careful. With the insistent rush of sexual desire, and all the imagined familiarity that went with it, they didn't have time to fall into a deeper, more sustainable form of love before they married, and I wonder now if they ever did.

When I was young and had learned a version of their story from my mother, I imagined my parents as a pair of thoughtful working-class pioneers, holding hands on the deck of the *Carinthia*, sailing away together after a long and steady courtship. But, in fact, the chronology proves the opposite. They quickly agreed to make a reckless leap without knowing where they would land. My mother was following her instincts. My dad was probably intoxicated by this surprising coalescence of circumstances and good omens. He had to leave quickly to escape two years of enforced army service, then suddenly there was a girl who'd go with him. And not just any girl. Marion was everything he thought of as beautiful and – more than that – she had the uncanny ability to read his innermost desires and then say them out loud.

It was a gift that I suspect became a curse.

My mother gave up a steady boyfriend when she met my dad, which led the rejected man to throw himself into a canal. He was rescued from the water by his friends, and I had always considered this element of the story to be a comic footnote. But if my mother had told him she was leaving imminently for Canada with a man she had met only a few days before, maybe his reaction was more understandable.

My dad told my mother during the voyage to Canada that the previous night he'd seen a UFO. It was for him a religious experience, in that it was final proof of his lifelong belief in the power of science fiction to come true. Without ever believing in fate, he was still willing to accept a celestial sign that he was about to fulfil his destiny.

45

'What did your mum and dad say?' Michael asked her.

The ship had finished turning and was moving steadily out towards the open sea. In a small steerage cabin, two cardboard suitcases stood side by side. His contained only a few shirts, his shaving kit, his degree certificate and the few books he was able to carry: a tattered copy of Ray Bradbury's *The Illustrated Man*, *The Stars, Like Dust* by Isaac Asimov and Arthur C Clarke's *Childhood's End*.

'Mum said do as you please, you're a free agent. I can't stop you. And Dad – well, Dad doesn't say much anyway. He said he hoped you'd be kind to me and he gave me a five-pound note. What about yours?'

'Canada might as well be on Mars as far as my mother's concerned, but she'll get over it.'

Michael put his arm over her shoulders and Marion slid her hand under his coat.

'Have you ever met anybody who's really, truly in love?' Marion said.

There was still a dance they had to do. He had said nothing yet about love.

'I don't believe so. Not the way you mean, I don't think.'

Obviously, he didn't believe in hearts-and-flowers emotions. Theirs was a practical arrangement. Surely she knew that? They were physically compatible. Their partnership was in both their interests.

'What about your parents?' she said.

'Well, my mum thinks a man who mends typewriters is some kind of a genius and my dad treats her like a household slave. Does that count?'

Marion held his waist, looking up to study his face again, storing away the tiny details. The mole on his cheek. The cleft in his chin.

'I'll bet your mum loves you to pieces. Especially so, you being the only one.'

'She thinks my shit doesn't stink, so you might be right. But that's only what she's – well, I suppose it's what she's evolved to do.'

'She must be so proud. Of you, I mean. Getting your science degree.'

'There's so much more than that I want,' he said, 'but I don't think I'll get the chance.'

He couldn't work out what it was about her but he found he was unable to stop himself from telling her the truth.

'Why wouldn't you, Michael? I believe you can do anything you put your mind to. You can be whatever you want to be. I just know it.'

It was as if she could see the wound. She could see it, raw, open and bleeding, and she didn't mind. She could even touch it without flinching.

'You don't understand, Marion,' he said. 'There are too many men like me out there already. They're all about my age. But they're all from la-dee-dah families and they went to the Right Kind of School. They were all drinking champagne and punting around Oxford and Cambridge while I was working nights to keep myself fed. Then, on top of that, I've wasted yet another year, so somebody might let me light Bunsen burners for school-boys for twenty quid a week. While those other men, they've been, well they've been . . .'

'Surely they should have been in the army, if they're young men?'

'Oh, it doesn't work like that, not for that kind,' Michael said. 'They got out quick, quicker than me, at any rate. To America or the Commonwealth. And they're the ones who are making science, making history. You know the expression "reaching for the stars"? Well, they've been actually reaching for the stars. Actually, literally, reaching for the stars. And that's where I should have been. Not with the dopes, left behind.'

'Where are you two headed for?'

Another passenger had joined them, leaning on the handrail.

'Montreal!' Marion said, laughing. 'One way.'

'So, what's in Montreal?'

'Michael's got himself a brilliant job,' she said. 'At a college there. It's like a university. He'll be teaching chemistry.'

'Well, congratulations! A young professor!' The man put out his hand and Michael took it. 'Which university?'

'It's Thomas More Institute. Not a professor, not just yet. And I'll be teaching other things, not just chemistry.'

A sudden increase in engine noise brought the conversation to an end and the man waved his hand over his head as he carried on unsteadily along the walkway.

✵ ✵ ✵

They sat up late on deck on their first night at sea, their legs touching under a pile of blankets.

'I like your middle name.'

'What, Harvey? I think it's an affectation. Nobody needs more than two names.'

'I don't think it's affected at all. It's old magic. It's supposed to protect you.'

'And how exactly would it do that?'

'A middle name is a secret. If fairy-folk know a baby's whole name they can steal it, then leave one of their own in its place.'

He leaned across and kissed her. 'I thought you might be a witch – it's probably too late for me now.'

Marion laughed. 'I can see your future, it's true. All mapped out, Michael *Harvey* Briggs.'

'So now you know my middle name, what magic are you going to do to me?'

'I think I'll wish it so you can never let me go.'

'I'm under that spell already,' he said.

'You'll never regret it,' she replied. 'I'll be your lucky charm.'

He held her close to him, resting his face against her neck to breathe in the warm scent of her skin.

'What did you mean, when you said you could see my future?'

'I heard what you said before about getting left behind. But I know you'll be famous. Whatever you do, the whole world will know it. And for years and years, people will talk about you and remember your name.'

'But you hardly know anything about me, not yet anyway,' he said.

'I don't need to,' she replied.

✻ ✻ ✻

After Marion had fallen asleep, Michael carried on looking up into the extraordinary infinite blackness. The wind had dropped and the sky was perfectly clear. All around him, above the ocean and reflected in its surface, Michael could see a whirl of galaxies. The quiet rhythm of the ship's engines mingled with the spectacle, giving sound and vibration to the universe in perfect motion. Out here, deep space objects he had only ever seen in books were visible: the Spindle in Draco, the Cat's Paw . . .

'You an astronomer too?'

The man had reappeared, standing under the safety light, smoking a cigarette.

'I know a bit – I've read quite a bit, that is. But to be honest, I've only ever seen the sky over Lancashire.'

The man looked up, then he threw the burning stub. It fell all the way to the water and went out.

'What your wife said about that college. I know the place and I wouldn't want you to be disappointed.'

'She's not my wife,' Michael said. 'At least, not yet. There wasn't time. And she gets confused about things: she's not academic, you see. She makes dresses. She doesn't really understand what I do.'

'She seems like a lovely girl – you're a lucky man.'

'Yes, I am. But she gets mixed up, I explain things to her then the next minute, it's gone.'

After the man had left, Michael wondered if he'd said too much and given himself away. He'd need to be more careful, now he had something to lose.

It was then that he noticed something hovering above the ship's wake. As he watched, he could see it had no wings of any kind, either fixed like an aircraft or in motion like a bird or a flying fish. It was still, in one position, as if suspended on invisible wires. Michael looked around quickly, wondering if there were any other witnesses apart from himself. Then he moved a few steps nearer, trying to work out if it was as close to him as it seemed. After a moment, it shot sideways and stopped abruptly, like a tiny silver carriage sliding to the end of a rail. It turned a white beam, like a single eye, towards his face, then began an erratic dance, slipping and turning, moving from point to point. Its persistent brightness carved a three-dimensional form in the air with swinging, parabolic strokes, at the centre of which, Michael realised, was – himself.

It is aligned with me, he thought, as it completed the shape and disappeared. It's been mapping my coordinates in spacetime. It knows where I am. It knows that I'm here.

He would tell Marion about it but no one else. At least, not yet. For now, it wasn't something a scientist should believe.

46

My mother's prediction was right, in a way. People do still know my dad's name because of what he did, though not for the reason he would have wanted. Oracles are prone to paradox and irony, and never say unambiguously what they really mean. My mother's mystical interventions were always sincere, and she intended them to be helpful, but prophecy is a dangerous business, often misconstrued as some kind of guarantee. And sceptics can be just as easily taken in as the credulous, if given a glimpse of their heart's desire and an easy path by which to get it.

My dad's rational self was surprisingly easily seduced by the possibility of magic, as is evident in his early infatuation with my mother and her all-seeing blue eyes. But then, he wasn't the first and is unlikely to be the last man to draw false courage from the coming together of an appealing prediction and a plausibly portentous event. A UFO fitted my dad's beliefs, just as horoscopes, cloud forms, answered prayers or tea leaves might suit the fanciful instincts of others. In an optimistic mood, anything might be interpreted as a good sign. In darker times, a snake and a toad might look like a warning.

47

'We watched *The Incredible Shrinking Man* together as kids, didn't we? On TV.'

'Oh, loads of times,' my brother says. 'I'm still terrified of spiders. But I got into science fiction because we saw that kind of thing. Like Dad, I suppose. But not books: for me, it was film and TV.'

'I've always thought *The Incredible Shrinking Man* was science fiction. But I watched it again recently. It's more about 1950s paranoia: what scientists might be about to do to us, not for us. In the 1950s, *The Incredible Shrinking Man* probably looked like the nuclear near future.'

'The same is true of *Godzilla*, though,' my brother says. 'Which is, I think, a sort-of irradiated dinosaur. And *Tarantula*: an irradiated spider, obviously. There's *Them*, of course. Irradiated ants. One of my favourites, *It Came from Beneath the Sea*, a gigantic, irradiated octopus—'

'That's just radioactivity or chemicals or whatever making monsters,' I say. 'The most frightening thing about *The Incredible Shrinking Man* is that there isn't a monster. There's nothing Scott can do but survive. There's no way of winning. Slowly but surely, it's science that shrinks Scott away.'

'Then there's *The Beast From 20,000 Fathoms*,' my brother says. 'Who is, I believe, woken up from hibernation by a nuclear explosion. *It Came from Beneath the Sea* was originally shown in a double bill with *The Creature with the Atom Brain*, about an army of irradiated zombies—'

'You aren't listening to me, are you?' I interrupt.

'Yes, I am. And you're right. Shrinking is more like an incurable disease, I suppose. More like radiation sickness, that you'd get with a nuclear war. *The Fly* is quite similar.'

'Scott's situation is frightening because we can see his shrinking is inevitable. After the Cuban Missile Crisis, nuclear war must have felt as if it could happen at any moment. Do you know the Ray Bradbury story, "There Will Come Soft Rains"?'

'No, I don't think so,' he says.

'It's about an automated house, after a nuclear attack. The house carries on doing its daily duties even though the people who lived there are now just four black smudges on the living room wall. But the house doesn't know. Every day, the house reads a poem aloud to them, "There Will Come Soft Rains". It's by a First World War poet called Sara Teasdale. The poem is about how nature will carry on regardless, after humans have annihilated themselves.

'*Not one would mind, neither bird nor tree,*
If mankind perished utterly;
And Spring herself, when she woke at dawn,
Would scarcely know that we were gone.'

'Blimey, that's gloomy,' my brother says. 'Give me an irradiated octopus anytime.'

48

In the summer of 1962, five years after their first date at *The Incredible Shrinking Man,* my parents were on another ocean liner. This time, they were sailing from New Zealand to the West Coast of America, heading for a new life near the Pasadena rocket site. The ship's captain announced midway that he'd decided to divert from their original course so the passengers could enjoy an unusual spectacle: it was a nuclear test explosion, taking place at Johnston Atoll in the North Pacific. My mother made herself a cardboard CND badge for the occasion, though she was probably more anti-war than anti-nuclear. She was as excited about the event as everybody else.

I hadn't ever considered whether this story was true, even though I'd heard it many times. It didn't really matter to me if it was. It sounded partly true – an embellished anecdote of my mother's from their early marriage with a kernel of fact somewhere inside it. But what my mother said she'd seen is corroborated by an article by journalist Gilbert King, published in 2012 in *Smithsonian* magazine. 'Going Nuclear Over the Pacific' is based on descriptions from other eyewitnesses who were there, on 9 July 1962. The Atomic Energy Commission created what it called 'the greatest man-made light show in history', 250 miles above the Pacific Ocean, with the detonation of a one-and-a-half-megaton thermonuclear warhead mounted on the nose of a Thor rocket. It was a hundred times more powerful than the Hiroshima atomic bomb and the explosion could be seen for thousands of miles. The view from Hawaii, Fiji and New Zealand was considered to be particularly good.

Afterwards, an aurora turned the moon blood red for several minutes. Clouds became black silhouettes, with the whole sky suddenly in photographic negative. Other observers described a vast, iridescent green ball and pulsing beams that rotated through the colours of the rainbow, like a celestial kaleidoscope.

Meanwhile, on board ship, there was a mushroom-cloud fancy-dress party on the viewing decks during the bomb blast, with a dance band and a buffet. King Neptune arrived at midnight, riding on a float pulled by seahorses and accompanied by an entourage of scantily dressed mermaids. There hadn't been a mushroom cloud of course, it was an aerial detonation, but mushroom clouds had already become the dominant symbol of the nuclear age. Very few people on board considered what the risks might be, standing in the open air watching a nuclear bomb going off. Like supernatural monsters, radiation clouds and toxic fallout were only scary in the movies.

My mother occasionally suggested that her unexplained hypercalcaemia could have been triggered by exposure to radiation. It had been a wasting disease, eating away at her bones, like futuristic illnesses tend to be in science fiction. She'd been to the rocket base in Pasadena when my dad was working there, where they did experiments to simulate the effects of radiation in space. But if it was radiation that nearly killed her, it was more likely to have been on their way to Pasadena, when they oohed and aahed, danced and drank under an electromagnetic thermonuclear blast, in the summer of 1962.

Maybe a sparkling chemical cloud had drifted towards her unseen, above the surface of the sea, winding itself around her as she stood on the deck. Maybe her husband had been somewhere else at the time. Maybe he had gone down to the cabin to fetch something, like Louise had done.

It would have been imperceptible, at first. But perhaps there was a moment when she, like Scott, had started to shrink.

49

My parents and infant brother moved to a modern duplex in nearby Altadena, California, before my dad started work at the Pasadena Jet Propulsion Laboratory sometime in the autumn of 1962.

JPL had started life as a project to develop safer liquid-propellant rocket engines, led by Hungarian mathematician and physicist Theodore von Kármán. He took his experiments out into the California desert in the summer of 1936, due to the risks to people and buildings from large explosions, settling in the Arroyo Seco just outside Pasadena. The programme was then purely military, in particular the development of guided missiles. But in 1962, JPL moved from army control to NASA, the newly created civil space agency. Earlier that year, NASA had also asked a university, the California Institute of Technology, or Caltech, to run JPL's projects, shifting the focus still further away from weapons research. When JPL's military character changed to something more like science fiction, recruitment expanded worldwide in the search for talented scientists who might want to go into space.

News of JPL's new mission statement reached my dad at the chemistry department of Victoria College, Wellington, in an advert in the *Biochemical Journal*, although it had probably taken some months to get to New Zealand by sea. It was an open invitation to apply to be in his boyhood fantasy: he might really go into space, be a spaceman and have a spacecraft. But the competition would be fierce for a job like this. He would have to beat the best of his generation, from Oxford and Cambridge, and Stanford, Harvard and Princeton. And Cornell, of course.

According to the advert, JPL's first mission, to be completed in 1963, was to soft-land the unmanned Surveyor spacecraft on the moon. It would collect samples of the lunar surface and put them in an electric oven, to break the material down and release gases into a molecule detector. These molecules would be the moon's elemental 'fingerprints', including any recognisable pre-life chemistry. The Surveyor programme was about to take off and look for the first clues to organic life elsewhere in space.

This is the probably the point, in early 1962, when my dad's curriculum vitae first started to peel away into fantasy, although the fake degrees were made sometime later.

According to the NASA archives, my dad went to work in Section 326, on imaginary space projects known as 'concept studies'. Soon after Surveyor's soft landing, the intention was for eight men to get into an orbiting spacecraft and go to Mars, just like they did in my dad's copies of *Astounding Science Fiction* magazine. His job was to work out the practical details – how exactly it was going to be done – using the best technological innovations that the early 1960s had to offer.

My dad often elided fantasy and reality – more than I previously appreciated, as it had turned out. But he was convinced that many things about space and time were just not possible yet, rather than being impossible. As a child, he'd once told me about an experiment he said he'd done on Mars called 'sticky string'. A weight on a string was thrown out and pulled across the Martian surface, through a culture which could grow any organic microbes it picked up. He said he'd discovered an unknown lifeform growing in the jelly, but he'd said nothing about it because the organism couldn't be categorised.

'It was, I think, silicon based,' he'd said in a matter-of-fact way. 'Rather than carbon, like we're familiar with here on Earth.'

I grew up believing that this had happened and was very disappointed when I found out nobody had ever been to Mars to do his sticky string experiment. I'd told a few people about my dad's discovery but thought it prudent not to mention it again as I must have misunderstood what he'd meant. Later still, I read the short story 'The Talking Stone' by Isaac Asimov, first published in 1955, in which a silicon-based lifeform suffers a work-related accident on a spacecraft and sadly dies from its injuries.

Despite my dad's highly developed imagination and his over-whelming desire for science fiction to come true, Pasadena turned out to be a dream that didn't last. Of all my parents' moves between occupations, communities and continents, the transition from California back to England at the end of the Pasadena episode, in the summer of 1963, is the hardest of them all to understand. Until this point, my dad's career had been on an upward trajectory, yet after a little less than a year, his next step seemed to have been from rocket science to agricultural feed, when he went to work for a Wiltshire firm called Analytical Laboratories.

As he was packing his bags to leave California, the first Mars probe launch would have been only a few months away. Surely it couldn't have been planned this way?

Maybe my dad gambled everything on a forged PhD as part of a pitch for a permanent job at the Jet Propulsion Laboratory.

If so, it would have been a dangerous strategy. He was trying to join a tight circle of space scientists in which there would be a high risk of being caught out by someone from the chemistry faculty at Cornell. The situation he'd left behind at the university in Wellington also had the potential to ruin his chances. Whether it had been blackmail or just striking a hard bargain, there was a lot of bad feeling about the Doctor of Science degree. Rumours about his character could have spread beyond the isolated scientific community in New Zealand and followed him to America.

It's always possible that Analytical Laboratories was a step up rather than a step down, for reasons that are hard to see at this distance of time. But what could Analytical Laboratories have had to offer him that NASA did not?

50

One of the reasons why I know so few hard facts about my dad's life, including what precisely he was doing between 1963 and 1966, is because there were only limited opportunities to find out.

When my parents separated in 1970 and my dad moved to Lusaka, Zambia, I was seven years old. I accepted the fact that he had always been some kind of scientist – 'biochemist' was the word most frequently used – and I was content to confabulate a story into any gaps if I needed to.

For much of the 1970s, my brother and I saw Dad about once a year, although we received picture postcards and air mail correspondence from around the world, suggesting increasingly frequently as time passed that we should be doing better at school. Dad would come to Europe for perhaps a week, maybe for a conference somewhere or a World Health Organization committee meeting. Then to England for two or three days, so we could spend about twenty-four hours with him in restaurants and department stores, at tourist attractions and in large hotels. We were allowed to eat whatever and whenever we pleased, in my case prawn cocktails and crème caramel at every meal.

Wherever we went, Dad told us unlikely things about the world, so it often felt as if we had rented a rowing boat on the Serpentine with Baron Munchausen, or visited a model village with Herodotus, followed by lunch in the dining car of a steam train on the Bluebell Railway. He always arrived with expensive gifts of a kind I realised much later were only sold in airports. For me, there were musical novelties, dolls in national costumes in stiff acetate boxes and Swiss watches. For my brother, it was chemistry sets, puzzles and robots.

I found my dad's superficially sunny disposition appealing and he seemed genuine to my childhood self. Looking back from adulthood, I can see that he used laughter to sidestep other people's emotions and what might have seemed like a funny invitation could just as easily be a warning. It was said at the time that I was sick whenever I saw him because I ate too much, and it's true that on the journey home I always ended up vomiting into a gutter.

Once I developed a voice that could be heard, I chose not to take part anymore in these queasy trips into the stratosphere. Not because I didn't want to see my dad but because I couldn't bear the inevitable rapid descent, splashing down in the same grey sea. It upset more than just my stomach.

When I was in my mid-teens, I relented and three times I stayed with him for holidays. I went to Australia in 1977 and 1982, and to Spain in the summer of 1986, the last summer of his life. As he always lived in the same kind of house wherever in the world he was, these were journeys into parallel versions of our childhood family homes. On these few extended visits, we'd play the parts of a father and a daughter to the best of our ability, but neither of us had much experience to bring to the roles and I don't think our performances would be thought of as credible. My character was an older version of the receptive audience I'd learned to be during his long absences, trying to absorb as much information as I could from him during brief episodes of exposure. He usually played a raconteur who sooner or later had the better of everyone. The only exception to this was when we watched films; then we became two more natural people engaging with something else. I didn't get to choose the films but I don't remember minding.

I was fourteen in July 1977, when I went to Australia in the summer holidays. When I arrived, my dad had just come back from a lecture tour. He'd bought some pirate videos from a market in Hong Kong – the newly released *Star Wars* and *The Island of Dr Moreau*. They'd been filmed covertly with a shaky hand from the back of a crowded and noisy cinema, so after a few minutes, we looked for something else to watch instead. My dad was an early adopter of all types of gadget and he'd bought the first Betamax home video system a couple of years before. I scanned along the handwritten labels on the shelf and pulled out a tape marked: '*The Incredible Shrinking Man*'.

'Mum says you went to see this on your first date. Is that true?' I asked him.

'Yes, it's true,' he said. 'At the Futurist in Lime Street. From what I remember, she didn't get it at all, she thought it was romantic! It had been a toss-up between that and *Quatermass*. The second *Quatermass*, the one about the alien meteorites. She might have liked it better.'

In the end, we settled on *2001: A Space Odyssey*. During the opening sequence, my dad described how he'd worked in Pasadena with science fiction writer Arthur C Clarke, emphasising how close they'd been by not using the 'C'. He and Arthur Clarke had shared similar views about space time and agreed that it was quite possible to have multiple selves in parallel universes.

Later on, during the journey to Jupiter, my dad revealed that he'd discussed the practicalities of travelling so far through space with the film's director.

'Black holes would behave like super-highways,' he'd apparently explained to Stanley Kubrick. 'Using black holes to bypass the otherwise impossible time it would take for a man to go to the other side of the solar system.'

As he said the words, what he was describing happened on the screen. Space traveller Dave Bowman's spaceship reached the event horizon, where it slid into a perforation in the skin of time. Then Bowman was inside a house, with versions of himself.

'Time is bent, you see. Or possibly stretched, it's arguable either way,' my dad said. 'So, in theory, Bowman's every possible self – at any point in his life – could be present in the same place, in the same room. He was looking for a monolith on the other side of the universe, but he's split apart and has ended up inside a kaleidoscope of himself.'

The room was silent, apart from the sound of Dave Bowman's assisted breathing. He'd grown old inside his spacesuit, on the far side of an intergalactic non-returning membrane. And despite the company of his other selves, or perhaps because of it, Dave Bowman seemed more completely alone than any person I'd ever seen.

51

For many years, I believed what my dad said about being involved in the making of the film *2001: A Space Odyssey*. Then, recently, long after he last said anything, I came to doubt that anything he'd ever told me about himself was true. But there were so many possible strands created by his known fabrications, so many parallel selves he had created, that the veracity of my dad's claims about Stanley Kubrick wasn't a particularly high priority.

It isn't very hard to look for evidence of anything in the electronic age. So, when I saw that *2001: A Space Odyssey* was on television, I half-watched the journey to Jupiter again while I tapped a few keywords into my phone.

In a remote corner of the Stanley Kubrick archive, some letters came to light. I visited them in September 2022, at the library of the communication department of the University of the Arts in London.

2 February 1966
MGM Studios, Borehamwood

Dear Dr Michael Briggs,
Stanley Kubrick is currently filming a motion picture entitled 2001: A Space Odyssey *at MGM studios in England. The original story for this film was written by Mr Kubrick and Arthur C Clarke. It is being shot in Technicolor and will be released worldwide by MGM in Cinerama early in 1967.*

THE SCIENTIST WHO WASN'T THERE

The film concerns itself with provocative philo-sophical and scientific themes. It revolves around the discovery on the Moon thirty-five years from now of the first extra-terrestrial artefact. It is determined as the story unfolds that this first evidence represents an intel-ligence whose origin was other than Earth and that it visited our Moon during the Pleistocene period.

If you are acquainted with Mr. Kubrick's earlier films (Dr. Strangelove, Paths of Glory) *and with Mr. Clarke's writings* (Childhood's End; Profiles of the Future) *you will understand that this is not 'another science fiction film', but a very carefully developed extrapolation of what may be the reality of just a few years from now.*

Technical advice has been obtained from widely diverse sources such as NASA, IBM, Bell Laboratories, Dupont, and Minneapolis Honeywell.

As a Foreword to the film we will have a series of eminent scientists discuss their views on the likelihood of our encountering extra-terrestrial intelligence, the possibilities of communications with cultures on other planets, and the probable cultural impact of the first extra-terrestrial contact.

The interview can be filmed at your place of work or other suitable setting and should not consume more than an hour of your time. The purpose of this letter is to seek your participation in this introduction. If you can make yourself available to these ends we will arrange a time and place most convenient to your schedule.

Keeping in mind the objectives of this Foreword, to
help the audience realise that the basic subject-matter of
the film is not fantasy but possible if not probable fact, I
hope you will be able to favour us with a positive response.
Most respectfully,
Hawk Films Ltd.

My dad had written back a few days later. The letter was on headed
notepaper and sent from his place of work, Analytical Laboratories in Corsham, Wiltshire:

I had heard of Stanley Kubrick's new film through
Frederick C. Ordway III, and I would indeed be most
interested in taking part in a brief interview for the fore-
word. Perhaps you could briefly outline in more detail
precisely what you had in mind for the contents of this
interview.
It is likely that one of our laboratories here could
be used as a suitable setting. I am enclosing one or two
reprints of Exobiology, *that set out some of my views*
on this subject, and that you may find of interest with
regard to determining the content of my contribution to
the foreword.
Yours sincerely,
MH Briggs DSc
Head of Laboratories.

The reprints my dad refers to are of *Current Aspects of Exobiology,*
the book at my brother's house. Frederick Ordway had been a

senior NASA official at the time. He'd befriended Arthur C Clarke, or Arthur Clarke possibly, many years before and then became a consultant on *2001: A Space Odyssey*. My dad must have met Ordway at the Jet Propulsion Laboratories in 1962, but how well they knew each other is open to question. My dad could have typed his name carelessly or perhaps he didn't know him well enough to realise that Ordway's middle initial was I, for Ira.

For the time I spent with them in the archive, the letters created a pleasing interrelationship between the three of us: me, my dad and Stanley Kubrick. But that feeling quickly faded. These were just more disconnected scraps about a father I hardly knew. I'd found some more entertaining trivia. Some more stuffing to push in the holes in my half-empty past.

52

I used to have no early recollections of my dad at all. Having a child myself in my mid-twenties suddenly brought back two vivid scenes that must have happened when I was only a few years old. I'd unhooked them from the delicate chain of memory because they didn't suit the style of the rest of it, but becoming a parent helped me put them back.

In the first, my dad is watching *Quatermass and the Pit* on TV. I can see myself standing just inside the door, in pyjamas and barefoot. I am half-asleep and beginning to cry.

Demons have been released from the ground by excavations around what looks like an unexploded wartime bomb in a London underground station, Hobbs End. Stories about satanic possession around Hobbs End seemed to be coming true, and when the creatures suddenly appear on the screen, they are nasty, sticky and locust-like. But most horrifying of all, they have horns and hooves. I believe they are real devils.

My dad lifts me up to sit beside him. He explains that it's only ignorance and superstition that makes the people in the story think these creatures are devils. They're really Martians, who crashed at Hobb's End in a spaceship, the metal object in the ground, millions of years before. They escaped from their own planet because it was dying. And they brought their superior alien learning with them to the ancient Earth. Despite their appearance, these creatures have their own community, their own society, their own hopes, dreams and affections.

After I have been calmed by reason, my dad takes me back to bed.

As he tucks in the edges of the blanket, he says: 'When you go to sleep, you might dream about the Martians, living happily together under a beautiful purple sky and two red moons, wishing on falling stars. You might fly to the other side of the solar system and walk around in one of their cities, although it would look very strange to you or me. Of course, the Martians will be just as surprised to see you as the people were in Hobb's End. Because they think they are the only intelligent life, living on the only exo-planet in the universe, just like we do. But when you meet them, you can tell them: there's really nothing to be scared of. Now you know we're there, we can be friends.'

Despite having some happy dreams about Martians, like many small children, I was still afraid of ghosts. In the second memory, I've woken from a nightmare and found my way again to the living room.

On the mantelpiece, there used to be a replica of an old weapon, a blunderbuss, on a wooden stand. My desire to have the blunderbuss for myself was well known to everybody in the family. As I cry inconsolably, my dad picks up a newspaper and pulls out a double page, rolling it between his hands into a long cone. Then he bends the narrow end of the cone around to make a handle.

'This is a blunderbuss,' he says as he hands it to me. 'You can shoot bad dreams with it.'

In this second encounter, my dad has created a magical object, when reason was unlikely to be sufficiently persuasive. He knew he had the authority to make me a weapon with miraculous powers, but what he created was also an icon in the religious sense. It was an everyday representation of a sacred ideal, the blunderbuss, ceremonially fashioned to work miracles in ordinary life.

In my dad's mind, reason trumped unreason. But faith is powerful, no matter how flimsy its foundations. When otherwise all seems lost, believing in magic must be the ultimate human paradox.

My mother isn't there in either of these memories. She must have been in hospital again.

53

'Something's been bothering me. And I've worked out what it is.'

'Hello, good morning,' my brother says. 'What is it this time?'

I had overlooked a surprising clue in Stanley Kubrick's letter. It wasn't the film, or the film director, or even Frederick Ordway III. It was the address.

'Don't you think it's strange? Dad was from Manchester. Mum was from Liverpool. They had no reason at all to go to Wiltshire. But that's where they went in 1963, from America.'

'I've never really thought about it. Did he have a job to go to?' my brother says.

'He did. The job would have to be better than NASA to be worthwhile, wouldn't it? But it was at an animal feed laboratory, called Analytical Laboratories.'

'If you say so,' he says. 'I'm not sure I ever knew what it was called.'

'The address is on the letters I showed you, from the Kubrick archive. It was near where we lived.'

'Near Chippenham, yes – so?'

'But it wasn't in Chippenham, though. It was in Corsham. Stanley Kubrick wrote to Dad in 1966 at Analytical Laboratories Ltd in Corsham. And Dad replied on the company notepaper from the same address.'

'Well,' my brother says. 'So what?'

'You know there are several years in the chronology, from 1963 to 1966, when we know almost nothing about what Dad was doing. There's something very odd about this job at Analytical. According to the patents register, Dad started applying for patents for animal feeds soon after going there, between 1964 and 1966. Not exactly what you'd expect after all the space stuff.'

'Can you patent animal feed?' my brother says. 'I thought cows ate grass.'

'And according to Companies House, there wasn't a company called Analytical Laboratories in those days. The only evidence that it existed at all is in the Kubrick letters.'

'Look,' my brother says, 'can't we just assume that there was a company called Analytical Laboratories where dad was working in 1966, otherwise Stanley Kubrick wouldn't have sent him a letter there? I don't know much about Stanley Kubrick but he makes very entertaining films, so I'm prepared to trust him on this one. And he got a letter back as well. So – QED.'

'That's not the point. Analytical Labs was sort of there but it had a different name. It was called the Berkshire Industrial and Chemical Agency. Later on, the company officially changed its name, at Companies House. Berkshire Industrial hadn't ever been agricultural at all. It was a quarrying company.'

'At the moment, I'm failing to grasp why any of this matters,' my brother says.

'Because back then, Corsham was a Ministry of Defence base. And when dad went to work in Corsham in 1963, it was the home of CGWHQ, the Central Government War Headquarters.'

'Forgive me, but were we at war in the 1960s?'

'The Cold War, stupid. CGWHQ was the national centre for Cold War preparations. Top secret at the time, obviously.'

'Well, obviously,' he says.

'The original project was codenamed "Subterfuge".'

'I see. This is all very Len Deighton.'

'Since when have you read any Len Deighton?'

'There's plenty about me you don't know, you know. I've seen *The Ipcress File*. I'm sure that's more than sufficient to have an opinion.'

'I knew you hadn't. Anyway, the CGWHQ was mainly under the ground. It was a small town inside a nuclear bunker, in a disused stone quarry. Hidden inside miles and miles of old mine workings.'

'OK,' my brother says. 'Let's recap. Whereas before, you thought our dad had a job in a cow food factory, it turns out now he was working in a kind of James Bond-style subterranean lair.'

'Something like that.'

'I was just checking I'd understood you correctly. Are you certain this isn't anything to do with your childhood obsession with Roger Moore?'

'It's nothing to do with Roger Moore, I promise. And it's quite possible he was doing both. Farming would need to adapt if there was a nuclear war, otherwise there wouldn't be any food.'

'That's assuming there's anybody left alive to eat it,' my brother says. 'Like in the poem.'

'I think the name Analytical Labs was a cover. Dad had been working on classified projects for the American government just before he got the job. He already had NASA security clearance.'

'True,' my brother says. 'He used to dress like an international man of mystery as well.'

'That summer when I went to Spain, he was rambling on a fair bit, about having affairs and stuff. But he also told me he'd done secret work for the government. With microfilm, and a gun.'

'He was very drunk, of course. Where is all this going?'

'I think there's another story about Dad. I think he really did do undercover work, at Analytical in Corsham, and maybe afterwards, when he was employed by Schering. It was something he was well qualified to do, for a change. We know from the research scandal, and now the fake degrees as well, that he was comfortable with pretence.'

'That's a nice way of putting it,' my brother says.

'He went to work for Schering, a German pharmaceutical company, at the height of the Cold War. With no good reason to be in that job, either. I think it all just adds up.'

'I'm only asking, but what difference would it make? Even if he was?' my brother asks.

'Well. I suppose I'd know the truth.'

'But the truth about what?'

I think for a minute.

'The truth about why he wasn't there.'

54

My brother and I grew up in front of the television. We watched it every day for as long as we could, and we watched anything. We'd watch it for the sake of watching it: it was a magic lantern, at the same time hypnotic and soothing. Our television set was left over from the old house, from our former life, so it was a huge piece of mid-century furniture, in a heavy teak cabinet with folding doors that closed across the screen. My mother chose it after reading George Orwell's *1984*, so it couldn't watch her when she wasn't watching it.

When there was nothing else on, we watched Open University modules and Trade Test Transmissions. These were short films that were broadcast for the benefit of television shops, who needed to tune in the new colour sets. We found them perfectly good entertainment, even though they were often unedited footage of gondolas or tropical fish, which we watched in black and white.

The first episode of *The Persuaders!*, an adventure series about an American millionaire and an English nobleman solving international mysteries, was shown on ITV shortly before my eighth birthday. Opinion was not in any way divided about which was the better performance, as nearly everybody who watched it at all preferred Tony Curtis's raffish Danny Wilde to the rather rigid and improbable Lord Brett Sinclair. But by 1971, I was already some way advanced in a lasting preoccupation with Roger Moore, which started with a set of core beliefs derived from intensive study of his character in *The Saint*. By 1971, I believed in Roger Moore, and that he sometimes appeared on television to demonstrate to the world the perfect qualities he possessed. Even his lack of charisma in *The Persuaders!* was probably a Christ-like act of self-sacrifice, to support a late resurgence in Tony Curtis's waning career.

I had pictures of Roger Moore everywhere in my room, and kept cuttings about his life, his movements, his habits and his interests. I sometimes drew pictures of him, with an authentically medieval lack of proportion or perspective. When a neighbour sent a note to my mother following a teatime visit, she made a point of expressing her gratitude for the wealth of information I'd provided about Roger Moore's parentage, his upbringing, his educational achievements and his troubled early marriage to Dorothy Squires. I think the neighbour had been trapped for some time in my company before help arrived. I was certainly the youngest and possibly even the only ever Roger Moore bore, and for several years I would discuss little else. The apotheosis of my Roger Moore worship was achieved when the James Bond film *Live and Let Die* went on general release in 1973.

James Bond as a film character already played a significant part in my pre-adolescent understanding of normal adult life and interpersonal relationships, even before *Live and Let Die*. The older films were shown on television, and because the plots were impossible for a child to follow, I assumed they were noisy and colourful anthropological lectures. With little to go on from my day-to-day experience through which I might interpret my dad's behaviour, he appeared to be very like 007. He was always getting on and off aircraft, he seemed to live in five-star hotels, he ate all his meals in restaurants and, in those days, there was little sign that he had anything as mundane as a domestic life. I added in a few details about his frequent trips to the World Health Organization using material from the TV sci-fi thriller *The Champions*. He could easily have been the fourth member of Nemesis, the United Nations law-enforcement agency whose agents acquired special powers after a plane crash in the mountains of Tibet. They often stood in front of Lake Geneva's Jet d'Eau, which was outside their office window, where I thought my dad must have stood himself when he was in Switzerland.

I saw *Live and Let Die* at the cinema in Leicester Square with my dad, on one of his brief and irregular visits to England. I had no idea what the film was about, only that Roger Moore was made manifest in it. The following week, I bought a set of tarot cards of the same design as Solitaire's.

It was many years before I made the connection between my childhood preoccupation and my dad's absence. I'd privately concluded that the reason why my dad wasn't there was because he was really an international playboy and a spy.

55

1963, Corsham HQ, Wiltshire

'Dr Briggs?'

'Please, call me Michael.'

Maybe he should talk to them about that, he thought. But this wasn't the moment.

'It's nice to finally meet you. How was your flight?'

'Oh, better than the boat, certainly. It was our first time on a 707. It took five days when we went the other way six years ago. To Canada.'

'A lot has changed since you were last here, Michael, hasn't it? The world is getting smaller every day. In some ways, anyway.'

'The weather hasn't changed that much, mind you. Still, we've had plenty of sun since we were last in GB.'

A woman came into the room and unplugged a percolator on the console table by the window. She made two cups of coffee and put them on the desk before leaving again and closing the door behind her.

'So,' he said. 'What is it that you want me to do?'

The man handed him an envelope.

'There's something inside there you should sign. But you don't need to worry about that now. You can do it at your leisure and return it to my secretary in the post. There's no magic in signing it, legally speaking. You just have to know it's there.'

Michael slid it into his inside jacket pocket.

'And now the formalities are over with, can you tell me about the work you were doing. In Pasadena?'

Michael took a sip of coffee.

'Well, I suppose we are all friends, aren't we? The truth is I was mainly working on scenarios for a crewed mission to Mars. Based around the Wernher Von Braun Project Plan. You know about Von Braun obviously, who defected to the USA. He designed the V2 rocket bomb, of course. Von Braun proposed that a thousand three-stage rockets could be launched from Earth carrying parts for a mission to an orbiting space station. Then we'd build ten spacecraft already in orbit, each one capable of carrying about eight men. Those spacecraft would then continue the journey to Mars. The astronauts will land themselves on the Martian surface in gliders. That's basically it.'

'And can you say how far advanced the work was on this project?'

'Well, I don't believe it would be giving away too many state secrets to say it's all still at the pencil and paper stage. There'll be an unmanned probe I should think, in the next couple of years. But Mars is a very long way away, you know.'

'So I'm led to believe,' the man said. 'But all in all, do you think your time at NASA has been productive?'

'Very much so. I hear on the engineering side they've got a pulse propulsion system that nearly works. Though the Nuclear Test Ban treaty is about to come in. So . . .'

'So, it will be impossible to do that kind of work anymore,' the man said. 'Which is a pity in a lot of ways. But necessary. You know, to put the brakes on internationally. With the Russians, I mean.'

'My area was biochemistry, the organic side. Strategies for detecting new forms of life. And for preserving the organic structures we already know about, of course. Astronauts for example.'

'I think that brings us on to the reason why you're here, Michael. The work we want you to do is also a concept study, very like the work you've been doing for NASA. But it is for a more imminent and serious challenge, and on a much bigger scale.'

'Go on,' Michael said.

'I should start by saying that the government's most pressing current concern, in private that is, is the escalating risk of a nuclear war. We have two main strategies to address that potentiality. We want to maintain the balance politically, so it doesn't happen. But if the balance is lost, we'll need to shelter as much of the population as we can, and as much of the fabric of civil society as we can, until . . . Well, I'm not sure until what, but that is the fall-back position. On the plus side, we've got a new detection system which will give us a comfortable four minutes' advance warning. But then again, four minutes isn't very long.'

'The same scenario was being discussed a fair bit at Caltech, so I'm not unaware of it,' Michael said.

'Until recently, despite what's in the newspapers getting worse and worse, nobody in power has been particularly concerned about the impact of all of this on public morale. The British public were stoical in the Blitz, no thanks to your Dr von Braun, of course. But things have changed. The Campaign for Nuclear Disarmament, the CND, is rattling a lot of people, making them less trusting of government to look after them.'

'We are now in the Space Age,' Michael said. 'Anybody who's read any Ray Bradbury or Arthur Clarke knows there's bound to be social upheaval.'

'Perhaps, perhaps,' the man said. 'But the concept study we have in mind is a kind of British nation in space. Where you were asked at JPL to look after the safety and wellbeing of eight men at a time in a spacecraft going to Mars, we would like you to imagine taking similar care of 53 million people, all at once. In a similarly radiation-filled environment. We want you to join the team that's working out how they'd breathe, eat, drink and cooperate. Whatever you think might be relevant.'

'And what would you use all this research for?'

'It would feed into the strategic plan. And an information campaign, one that will encourage a positive attitude.'

'To nuclear war?'

'Well, to the government's response. We want the Cold War strategy to appear modern and forward-looking. More like science fiction, in a way.'

'When do you want me to start?' Michael asked.

'As soon as you like. In terms of what you might say to friends and family, we recommend soft-pedalling what you do. Wiltshire is a farming county. We usually say that the work at Analytical Labs is at the agricultural end of chemistry, which is to some extent true.'

'It doesn't sound very top secret though, what you've asked me to do. Why all the cloak and dagger?'

'It's less to do with where you'll be working and more who you'll be working with. There are government ministers involved and if the balloon goes up, they'll be coming here, to Corsham. Come with me. I'll take you on a tour of HQ before you go off house-hunting.'

56

During the time my dad was Analytical's head of laboratories, from 1963 to 1966, he registered four international patents for scientific products, three of them for synthetic animal feed using polymer gels.

The fourth patent, registered in May 1966, is different from the other three:

A feed for young ruminants comprising a normal ruminant feed having lyophilised rumen fluid incorporated therein. The fluid may be obtained from the rumen of slaughtered ruminants, or via a chronic fistula.

'That sounds pretty disgusting,' my brother says. 'What's "lyophilised rumen fluid"?'

'According to Google, it's freeze-dried digestive fluid from the first stomach of a cow or sheep.'

'And I know I'll regret asking, but what is a "chronic fistula"?'

'It can be a tunnel in the flesh due to disease, connecting things together that aren't normally connected. But I don't think that's what he's talking about. I think these fistulas are intentional. To drain rumen, then keep the drain open artificially. In a living animal. Like a tap.'

'A tap in a cow? Why would anybody do such a thing?'

'I think it was a technique that was already being used in animal feed laboratories. But not to make the animal feed itself.

What all these patents have in common is they're ideas for new foods to replace the natural things sheep and cows might eat. Like grass. I think these patents envisage a situation where you have sheep and cows, but no grass.'

'This supports your theory about Cold War research,' my brother says. 'And it also explains why I remember him having a cow with a hole in it.'

'The holey cow! See how it all fits? When there's no grass for sheep or cows after a nuclear strike, when the land's poisoned, I think these patents were for Cold War farming R&D. If the plan was for the whole government and half the civil service to go underground in Corsham, which we know it was, then they needed to get some basic farming down there.'

'We've established that our dad was a fantasist and a fabricator of qualifications,' my brother says. 'But he did actually work on a Mars probe. From what you say, he also did actually invent novel forms of space food for farm animals, using a holey cow. Then he did actually make a handbrake-turn into synthetic hormones for humans, at Schering. This is very far from being a natural career path, isn't it?'

'That's exactly why I think government secrecy is the missing link between the last two things,' I reply.

'Anyway,' my brother says, 'didn't that whole "feeding dead sheep to cows" thing turn out to have been a very, very bad idea?'

'You mean BSE? One of Dad's favourite subjects when we were younger was Creutzfeldt-Jakob disease, of course. Do you remember? He used to call it the rarest disease in the world. Before everybody else started talking about it.'

'Are you going to pin that one on him as well?' my brother says.

57

Between 1963 and 1966, it's plausible that my dad was working for the government at the Corsham Cold War Headquarters. He was at the time a biochemist with interests including crabs' eyes, woodlice, H G Wells and meteors, with a strong conviction that he might very well know all science.

But he'd been given the highest possible level of security clearance and had worked for the United States government on classified research. While the USA had recently joined with Britain in a Cold War resistance pact, the Special Relationship, so it should have been sharing information, a British scientist with inside knowledge of NASA's policies and projects would have been of significant interest to the British government.

Nobody yet knew what space might add to the Cold War. But it was a resource to be dominated, and potentially a new theatre for direct conflict.

Any Cold War plan would have to include a nuclear attack response strategy, to meet the catastrophic biochemical effect of radiation fallout on ordinary citizens. This was an area of research in which NASA was already very far ahead.

58

'Was it Vladimir Putin who said, "There's no such thing as a former KGB man"?'

'Probably,' my brother says. 'Your point being?'

'Well, do you think the same thing applies to all kinds of covert government work? That once you've signed the Official Secrets Act, you never leave?'

'James Bond never retires, I suppose. Or Secret Squirrel.'

'The thing is, if I'm right about Dad, working for the government on the Cold War stuff in the early 1960s, then what might that tell us about what he did next, and why he moved on?'

'I can't believe doing secret things in this country is anything like being in the KGB,' he says. 'It's all Camp coffee, custard creams and tightly furled umbrellas, isn't it?'

'Georgi Markov was killed with a poisoned umbrella,' I say.

'That wasn't us though; it was the Bulgarians, probably.'

'Can we really be so sure?' I say.

'I think you're drifting into conspiracy theory, there. That way madness lies,' my brother says.

'That's the problem with this version of Dad's story, though. It's all too much like a sci-fi thriller.'

'Only if you want it to be,' he replies. 'I don't mind personally if he was just a perfectly ordinary dishonest scientist who made animal feed then hashed up some research about contraceptives.'

'Don't forget about space.'

'Yes, space, space – who could forget about space? The way he and Mum went on about it, you'd think they were in Pasadena for decades. How long was it really?'

'I think it was about ten months, not more than twelve. And that brings me on to my next point. Schering Chemicals, as it then was. Why do you think they gave him such an important job? He really wasn't qualified for it, even without knowing his doctorate was made up.'

'Oh, I don't know. It was the 1960s. He sounded like he knew what he was talking about, even though maybe he didn't. They took it at face value when he told them he knew all science.'

'It's easy to see why he would have wanted the job, of course. It was prestigious and I'm sure it was very well paid. Synthetic hormones were becoming the "next big thing". But I think there was something else, to do with Schering as a company. It may have been no accident that he went specifically to Schering.'

'You do know that "may have been no accident . . ." is quite a tinfoil hat turn of phrase.'

'I've been reading around, about Schering,' I say. 'It's an interesting company. They made lice powder and penicillin during the war and had some connection with the Nazis that they've had to live down since 1945. Then Schering decided to stay in Berlin after the wall went up in 1961. It was the only big company that didn't get out. They had a large factory and a development lab inside the GDR. When Dad went to work for them in 1966, Schering was a multinational chemical firm with one foot on either side of the Berlin Wall.'

'Are you saying that Dad was a government spy at Schering?'

'Maybe. But if he was, it wasn't Schering they were interested in. As far as I know, Schering was totally above board. The problem wasn't Schering. It was Jenapharm.'

59

Along with the story about the snake and the toad, my dad told me a few months before he died that he'd taken microfilm and a gun into East Berlin. And like the snake and the toad, it didn't make any sense at the time. I wrote it off as something he'd probably seen in a movie.

Between 1966 and 1970, my dad went to Berlin on business many times. He was responsible for the research output of Schering UK, so they could make and sell synthetic human hormones all around the world, in contraceptives and in Primodos. Schering's head office was in easy walking distance of the Berlin Wall crossings, including the most famous, Checkpoint Charlie. Café Adler was nearby, on the corner of Friedrichstrasse, where curious visitors to West Berlin went to watch the partition in action, and the armed border guards that patrolled it. My dad's job brought him into contact with people whose covert knowledge of the inner workings of the East German state would have been of high value to Western governments. And he could easily obtain permission to travel.

Schering maintained its connection with the East German pharmaceutical market from 1961 until reunification in 1989. The East German secret police, the Stasi, kept extensive files about Schering staff, some of which have been released into the public domain. We know that unnamed Schering executives frequently went in and out of the GDR, apparently on business.

Schering got involved in legal disputes about patents and licences in the East German courts, but only so they could protect their rights around the highly lucrative hormone products that they were selling elsewhere in the world. Schering was banned from selling its oral contraceptives in the GDR because the only supplier of synthetic hormones inside East Germany was the state-controlled company Jenapharm. Jenapharm was suspected by Schering of patent infringement and industrial espionage. After the reunification of Germany in 1989, Jenapharm was privatised and acquired by one of its international competitors: Schering AG.

My dad knew about pharmaceutical patents as he'd registered several in his own name. This part of Schering's business strategy would have been of great interest to him. Schering also organised clinical studies inside the GDR, despite having no products in the East German medicines market. At that time, there was no legal requirement for East German patients to give any form of consent if they were given experimental drugs. Between 1960 and 1982, Schering carried out several major synthetic hormone trials in East Germany, perhaps intended to show the GDR government the benefits of using Schering products. Jenapharm pushed back against any suggestion that external suppliers could get licences to protect its closed market in pharmaceutical products.

Decades later, it was revealed that, from 1964 onwards, Jenapharm was secretly producing anabolic steroids to be administered to East German athletes in a state-run doping programme. This was frequently done without the athletes' knowledge or consent.

Between 1966 and 1970, Schering's research directors went into the GDR and met with government officials, as well as members of the public who acted as research subjects. They would have encountered their counterparts at Jenapharm, whether in arm's-length negotiations or in closer discussions about matters of mutual interest. Schering also needed to keep a firm base in East Germany to monitor new Jenapharm products that might infringe its product designs.

During the four years when my dad was a senior scientist at Schering, he must have known about synthetic hormone research projects in East Germany. After he left in 1970, he had professional relationships with several pharmaceutical companies, including as part of the research that resulted in the 1986 scandal.

In the *Sunday Times* articles, journalist Brian Deer could only think of one reason why my dad was unable to explain where all the raw data had come from for his published studies of contraceptive risks. He must have dreamed it all up. But there is another possible explanation.

The man Brian Deer interviewed in Spain in the summer of 1986 was drunk and starting to crack. He said he didn't want to 'drop people in it' but it was never clear what he meant by that. If he wasn't solely responsible for the fraudulent research published in his name, then who else could have been involved?

In the early 1980s, the GDR was starved of international currencies and needed to get hold of sterling or American dollars. It has been suggested that several pharmaceutical companies bought East German research data with cash, to use in their own product development or marketing. If that was the source of the figures he used, then my dad would have struggled to explain this. There might really have been large cohorts of female research subjects – but in East Germany, unregulated and unprotected by rules around consent. These research subjects were probably unusually cooperative because they had little choice but to do what they were told or because they never knew they were in the research at all.

It's all just conjecture, of course. It's just as likely that, out of arrogance or laziness, my dad made up the data he needed based on other people's figures, as Brian Deer said. Then he got caught because he made the numbers too perfect to be true.

The Berlin Wall came down three years after the Deakin research scandal and my dad's death. Its secrets and spies now appear quaint and, apart from a few Cold War thrillers, are largely forgotten.

60

'I think I've finally solved it,' I say. 'My Cold War spy mystery, that is. It all fits. After Dad left Pasadena, he was a Cold War scientist, in the bunker in Corsham. Then he did a bit of spying in East Germany, probably for the government.'

'That doesn't sound completely incredible,' my brother says. 'I'm not sure if spying is a good or a bad thing. And as you said before, I suppose skulking around Berlin with a newspaper with a hole in it would have been a good reason why he wasn't there.'

'I really do think it's true.'

'Not just your Roger Moore fetish, then.'

'There is evidence,' I say. 'Even though it's circumstantial. But that's hardly surprising as it was all over years and years ago. It was supposed to be secret. And everybody who might have known about it is dead.'

'Well, as long as you're happy, that's the main thing,' my brother says. 'Though I do wonder if you're still looking for a better explanation than you're ever likely to get.'

I don't reply.

'You could just decide that it was nobody's fault that he wasn't there,' my brother goes on. 'That there was no pattern, no plot. Maybe it was just what happened to us. Because Dad doesn't have to have been a spy to have loved you. Or us. Just as not being a spy wouldn't prove that he didn't.'

'But what if he was a spy?' I say. 'What if he had a whole secret life, we knew nothing about?'

'Do you want my honest opinion?' my brother says. 'I think: so what? I think our dad was just young, and he was thoughtless, and selfish. Like we all are, sometimes. He was so busy chasing after what he wanted that he didn't think about the consequences for other people. So, the only love he had to give to us wasn't up to much. That's all it was. We were two little kids with no dad. And a mum who was a bit crazy, so there were times when we had to fend for ourselves. And sometimes we didn't do a very good job and things went wrong. We were let down. That's it.'

'I don't want that to be true,' I say.

'I know you don't. It's a sad story and you don't like sad stories,' he says. 'I don't either. It's another thing we have in common.'

61

'Saying our mum was just mad does hide the fact that there was a good deal more to her than that. Did I ever tell you the story about Mum and my therapist?'

There have been natural fluctuations in family life over the years when I saw my brother much less than I do now. But otherwise, my brother has been putting up with the sound of my voice without complaint since I was two years old, when I first started speaking.

'No, I don't think you did,' he says.

'It was about a year after Dad died, so it was 1987, when I was about twenty-five. I started having panic attacks. I felt like throwing up all the time, in public places and in crowds. I always had carrier bags in my pockets in case I was sick.'

'I do remember that bit,' he says.

'Anyway, somebody recommended this therapist, Vincent. Vincent had a previous career as a screenwriter, when he wrote scripts for sci-fi shows on TV, like *The Prisoner*. And spy stuff as well, like *Man in a Suitcase*.'

'So, Dad would have liked him,' my brother says.

'Vincent helped me to do some empty chair stuff, about Dad.'

'Which is?'

'It's a way of talking to somebody who isn't there. The empty chair in the therapy room is where they would have sat. I said some things to Dad about how I felt and I imagined what he might have replied. But that was all based on what I knew then, not what I know now. After about six months, I felt a lot better. So I stopped going for a while. I went round to see Mum and I told her about how well I was doing.

'"Do you know," she said, "I think some therapy might help me too. Can you give me his number?"'

'I'm getting a bad feeling about this,' my brother says.

'She forgot to ask me again, but she got his number anyway, out of the phone book. When I went back a few weeks later, she was in a very cheerful mood.

'"I've seen Vincent," she said. "But after the first session, we decided next time to go to the pictures instead."'

'Ah.'

'"Ah" indeed. They went to see *Les Liaisons Dangereuses*.'

'God almighty,' my brother says. 'But surely he shouldn't have done that?'

'The thing is, I didn't blame him at all, I still don't. Because I know what Mum was like. That's why I didn't want her to meet him in the first place. I knew she'd charm him, if she wanted to. Then she'd bamboozle him with her Gypsy Petulengro fortune telling and witch-traps in pebbles.'

'You always had more time for all that bollocks than I did. Did he have any obvious warts she could buy off him?'

'Both of our parents were hustlers, weren't they? In their own ways, and probably not intentionally, but still. I didn't want Vincent to like my mother more than me, which was childish. He wasn't really my therapist anymore, though I'd probably have gone back if they hadn't got romantically involved. I suppose I thought: she's probably lonely, and he's an interesting man of a similar age, so.'

'So?'

'So, I said nothing. I assumed she must have considered the consequences before she crossed that line. Presumably she'd decided that her connection with this man was of such significance that my feelings were less important. I avoided her for a while. When I saw her again, she told me she'd stopped seeing Vincent ages ago.'

'Why?' my brother asks.

'She said he wasn't very good in bed.'

62

My dad deceived my mother with an affair, probably for years. And possibly more than one. He told me in Spain that he'd had at least one previous affair, including a liaison with a woman who was by then in the public eye. Who knows if that was true or not. I'll add it to the list, anyway.

My dad announced one evening that the marriage was over then he disappeared, leaving my mother scrolling back through the screenplay of their life together. Previously unreleased extra scenes now explained the arguments, the unexplained absences, the indifference, the chance remarks and the hurried telephone calls. Her happier memories became a bitter catalogue of cruel tricks and the raw material for private jokes whispered behind another woman's hand. Poisoning my mother, if that's what he did, might have been the lesser betrayal of the two.

In the empty chair game in 1987, I played the part of a little girl who'd lost her daddy. This child was calmed and reassured by another man, who was in a way an idealised projection of the one I had lost.

I learned a sharper lesson when my mother used sex to beat me at an altogether different game. I'd seen this kind of power play before, so I shouldn't have been surprised to see a woman take a man from another woman, even when it was my own mother stealing my therapist. From everything I had seen and heard in childhood, I knew my dad had been lured away and that sexual desire had baited the trap. I learned at my mother's knee, as it were, that sex is a strategic weapon of war. And everybody is fair game.

The other woman in my childhood psychodrama had played her part exquisitely, according to type. This second wife was a winner, so my mother and me, we were losers. According to their fairytale reputation, stepmothers know that the battle is only won when what went before has been completely erased. Although, a sustained propaganda campaign, devaluing and undermining the past, could be just as effective. As a child, I perceived in my dad's wife a theatrical show of welcome with insidious undercurrents of spite: *It's not your fault, Michael but your children are lazy. It wouldn't matter so much if they were more like you but they aren't. They're very ordinary. Are you sure they're worth any more of your time, or your money?*

What I now know, so many years afterwards, throws a different light on my dad's relationships. At twenty-two, he'd married a local girl but he already knew his native town would never be the world for him. He was also morally weak, with an unprincipled belief that he was entitled to have anything he wanted. He pretended to be more than he was, successfully at first, but then his marriage to my mother became a stark reminder of everything he was trying to escape. In the next woman, he saw his own reflection, a mirrored counterpart of the person he believed he should have been.

I'd previously thought of my dad and his second wife as a golden couple, though I saw them through envious eyes and most of the time from a great distance. She was a doctor, he was a successful biochemist, and together they travelled the world, making science. They seemed to me to have all the money in the world; they had beautiful houses in sunny places, shiny cars and swimming pools.

Questions were asked in 1986 about how much of my dad's research was in fact the product of this husband-and-wife collaboration; his scientific fraud might not have been a highly lucrative sole enterprise but the stock in trade of a mom and pop store. My dad closed this idea down during the long interview in Spain in the summer of 1986: 'It's me that you want,' he'd said. 'Leave her out of it.' At the time, that sounded gallant. Maybe this protective impulse was genuine. Or maybe he didn't want to admit that his work was not exclusively his own, no matter how bad the reason was for standing alone in the spotlight.

This implied confession may have been the first sign that my dad's facade was crumbling, for reasons he successfully concealed from Brian Deer's scrutiny. Deer had access to Dr Jim Rossiter, the man who had guessed the truth about my dad's Cornell degree during the Deakin investigation. But, even then, the real story never came out: that my dad was not just a perpetrator of fraud, he was himself a fake. I've wondered since whether my dad's wife ever knew that she was married to a man whose elevated reputation was in fact built on pretence. It would have been to her an unbelievable suggestion, after everything he'd done. This was the secret he ended up protecting until death, and beyond.

In 1986, he'd have risked exposing that secret if he'd taken legal action against the *Sunday Times*. But left unchallenged, the *Sunday Times* story would have destroyed him anyway. There must have been a moment when he saw his parallel futures: versions of doing something or doing nothing, but all leading to the same inevitable outcome. Ruin.

Maybe it happened after the meeting in London. Or maybe it was later, on the journey home to Spain. But I've always believed that 26 September 1986, the day when I last saw my dad, was the day when he started to die.

PART 4

A Shrinking Man

Like one, on a lonesome road, who
Doth walk in fear and dread,
And, having once turned round, walks on
And turns no more his head;
Because he knows a frightful fiend
Doth close behind him tread.

Victor Frankenstein,
Recalling 'The Rime of the Ancient Mariner'
by Samuel Taylor Coleridge

Louise: I love you; don't you know that?
Scott: You love Scott Carey – he has a size and a shape and a way of thinking. All that's changing now.

The Incredible Shrinking Man

63

Friday, 26 September 1986, late evening

Michael stands on the rough track outside Villa Valencia while the taxi makes a scraping turn, then lurches away. He watches the lone beacon of a single brake light as it charts a steep, zigzag descent through the blackness, before disappearing into the far-off constellation of Puerto Banus.

His shirt sticks more firmly to his back and another wave of sickness washes over him, feeling more each time like dread. He's now in no doubt that something terrible has got inside his world and that it intends to destroy him.

He'd known it was there for some time, but without being able to sense how close it was or when it would finally show itself. Then, earlier that day, he thought he'd felt its breath on his neck. Then he'd heard its voice in his head. Then he'd recognised its face, momentarily at the window. Alone on the dark road, cold-blooded night creatures are whispering unseen among the heated stones. He twitches at each sound, each unhuman crawl and slither, but when he turns there's nothing there. He picks up his bag and hurries to relative safety, beyond the gate, inside the chain-link perimeter fence.

Michael sighs deeply as the door slams firmly shut behind him. Inside, it's perfectly quiet. He knows he has the house to himself. She won't be back until morning, which is something, at least. He has time. Only a little more time, but some time, in which he can think. He turns on the lights in the hall and cast iron chandeliers hanging high above him throw their shadows upwards into the vaulted ceiling. Bad spirits like dark corners, he thinks to himself; he could end up seeing things, if only the unbidden projections of his own imagination. There seemed to have been one haunting today already and he doesn't want there to be others.

At the other end of the long passageway, he reaches for the switch and the living room appears, illuminated. Vast ornamental mirrors face the glass doors to the terrace from each of the internal walls. They magnify the brightness and hold within themselves an infinite number of other near-identical living rooms. His panic is subsiding and supernatural concerns give way to an underlying, insistent thirst. Everything he wants is laid out on a silver tray on the table, apart from ice. He doesn't need ice. He swills orange bitters around in the bottom of a large glass then adds enough gin to create a plasma-pale wash. He puts the bottle aside unstopped without returning it to its place, rinsing the liquid around in his mouth as he pulls off his tie and throws it into a nearby chair. Then he takes a further gulp before he fumbles open the buttons of his sweat-soaked shirt.

So.

Inner warmth balances his outer discomfort, calming him further and reviving his senses.

What should my opening gambit be? He thinks.

A simple statement of fact, perhaps. It's legal advice, after all. There's nothing emotional about it.

But what, then, will she say?

Well: why, probably.

'Why?' he says loudly, projecting his voice towards the reflection on the far wall. He studies himself inside the other room, over there. Its milky white show-home walls are the same. Its chalk-washed furniture is gathered around clear glass tables in the same way, in silent conversation sets. The polar white fur rugs are the same, punctuating the same expanses of translucent white porcelain. This room is the same as it has always been, but he's never seen it this way, or himself, so looking-glass inverted.

It's very strange, he thinks. It's still my room, only I'm on Jupiter.

But she won't just say 'why?', will she?

She'll say: 'Why in God's name would he say that?'

That's when she'll appear in one of the doorways behind him, from the kitchen, perhaps, or the bedroom.

'Why would your barrister say such a thing? Why does he think we'll lose?'

He leaves Jupiter behind to walk around and think, while his glass is endlessly refilled by an invisible sommelier. But it's so hot. I thought it would be cooler inside, he thinks. But it's so hot. It's the middle of the night and it's sweltering. He throws open the doors to the garden but it brings no relief. A gentle, tropic wind dusts his damp skin with a film of salt and desert sand. He can see the black lawns beyond the balustrade are in a thermal form of darkness, radiating the heat from the day. On the surface of the swimming pool, the colourless reflection of the lights from the house makes cut-out silhouettes of the cultivated palms and orange trees.

There's a satellite blinking on and off in the sky above the blue-black Sierra Morena, moving towards a thin crescent moon.

Not a flying saucer, then. Not this time.

'Well, that's lawyers for you, I suppose, isn't it?' he says with a smile.

'And anyway, he didn't say we'd lose. He just said he didn't think I'd win, that's all.'

She would never let it go at that, surely not.

Nobody would.

'But you said. You told me – you said you could stop all this legally. You said suing the papers couldn't possibly go wrong.'

She would come towards him then, subtly changing her tone. Touching his shoulder. Brushing his neck momentarily with the tip of her finger.

'You promised me,' she'd say.

Had he? Had he really promised her?

Michael pushes his hand into the front pocket of his trousers, allowing his thumb to stroke the smooth shape of his wedding ring. He feels it begin to loosen and slip out of position, before rolling easily over his knuckle.

He traps it quickly in a fist. And it slides back.

I couldn't have promised that, could I? How could I possibly have promised that?

He becomes aware of the pungent scent of warm citrus, drifting in from the garden.

Where honey-bees hum melodies
And orange trees scent the breeze.

What was it that Marion had said?

Even when Scott is so small he lives in a doll's house. Even when there's no hope of them ever having a normal life again. None of it matters. That's what love really is.

'I think we should listen to him anyway,' he says to the empty room, drawing himself back into the present. 'He's trying to help us. To help me. To – well, you know. Do the right thing.'

He can picture her easily, now. Leaning back against the arm of a chair, with her hands clasped in front of her.

She's humming to herself. Then she's singing.

I want to be a home sweet home-er,
There I'll settle down . . .

He knows this voice so well. But it isn't a sound. It's a very distant memory.

'Oh Michael,' she says to him suddenly, suppressing a giggle. 'You do know you're going to have to see this through to the bitter end. Don't you?'

There isn't really a choice anymore. There's no other option. It was always bound to happen this way, anyway.

'I've told you, years ago. It's your destiny.'

He wants to answer her, but he's more mixed-up than he realised.

'Did you get a chance to see your daughter, in the end?' she says.

Did she say 'your daughter' or 'our daughter'? He isn't sure.

'Yes. Yes, we had lunch together. She's – you know. Still wasting her time. Doing nothing.'

'It's such a pity, isn't it. That she isn't more like you.'

'Well, maybe,' he says.

When he opens his eyes again, he's leaning against the wall and she's no longer there.

Seeing ghosts again? he says, shaking his head to clear the image, moving the coloured shards in the kaleidoscope until they settle.

This isn't like you. Not like you at all.

'There was more of gin than djinn about her I think,' he says to the almost-empty bottle.

Nonetheless, his wife is going to have to know, and soon, why they have no options left at all.

No good ones anyway.

Well, you see, my darling, he thinks he might begin. There are one or two things I haven't mentioned, about who you think I am. Because, the thing is, I haven't been entirely truthful.

'The fact is,' he says out loud, 'there are things about me, about the past, that I don't want to go into. And I would have to go into them, I'd be asked all sorts of questions about those things, if it all went in front of a judge. So, I'm afraid I just can't do it.'

This speech is not bad. But it lacks an obvious focus.

Then he remembers the books.

The books! The books.

The blue one and the red one. If I get out the books, then we can sit down together, like reasonable people, and I can show her what I did. How I tore off the old blue covers. How I had them made all over again, with new gold letters on the outside. And the red one: well, the red one didn't really exist in the first place. I made that one from scratch. I can show her that the red one is almost empty, with only a few fading photocopies inside. Maybe she'll understand, when she knows why I had to do it. She might even admire my creativity.

Michael makes his way unsteadily to his study, keen to try out the strategy straight away. He goes behind his desk and he reaches up to the shelf.

While he is on his way down the long corridor inside Villa Valencia, Michael is also walking along the Embankment, still trying to take in the lawyer's advice. This Michael is on a busy London street, a thousand miles away. He turns up his suit collar against a sudden chill and he pushes his hands into his pockets. The Thames flows beside him, oily and thick, like the city river of his childhood, its surface shimmering with artificial light and unbroken by the currents underneath. He rubs his wedding ring absently with his thumb.

Back in a book-lined office on the side of a Spanish hill, Michael reaches up to the shelf, but there's nothing there. In the space where they should have been, there's nothing. The blue and red theses have gone.

But they haven't gone though, Dad, have they? They were never there. They never got to Spain. Don't you remember? You left them behind in your office at Deakin. You must remember, surely? Because of the snake and the toad?

He feels along the empty shelf with his fingers, not quite able to believe the evidence of his senses. But there's only a paperback book, worn at the edges, lying on its side.

He takes down his old copy of *The Illustrated Man* and turns it over in his hands.

Michael also stands still, blocking the busy pavement by Temple tube station.

Where are they?

Dad, the registrar in Australia has got the red and blue books. He's going to send them to you, in a parcel, with a note.

It's starting to rain and a crush of city commuters pushes him momentarily off his feet. His pulse is racing and he feels a rising chill of nausea.

Where on earth are they?

I just told you, Dad. Listen to me. The registrar will send them to you. But by the time they arrive – I'm so sorry, Dad. You'll already be dead.

64

Tuesday, 26 September, 2023

'What do you think it's like? When you realise there's nothing you can do, that something terrible is coming to get you, and know you can't get away?'

'You're talking about Dad.'

'I saw Dad get on a train, just any old train to London. And then he was dead. And I never saw him again. His situation was already disastrous, looking back, because now we know there was no way he could ever have recovered. Not professionally, personally, financially, not in any way. He was a hollow man, waiting to get found out and taken to the cleaners. But was there a moment when he just suddenly knew it was all over? Or do you think it was more like in a cartoon. Like when Wile E Coyote runs off a cliff and he's in the air, but he doesn't fall straight away. Not until he looks down and sees that the cliff has gone.'

In 1986, my brother and I had been in our twenties. We led very different lives from each other in those days. But between the *Sunday Times* article in September and the phone call two months later, we had something unique in common. We were how we used to be, when our childhood bedrooms were side by side. We didn't know what was happening to our dad but without knowing it, he'd brought us together.

After it was over, we drifted back into our parallel lives. We functioned together as siblings when we had to look after our mother, particularly as she grew older and more frail. We marked the cycle of gift-giving anniversaries. From time to time, we walked our dogs together. We've never lived very far apart and looking back, I think I liked to know he was nearby, as I had done when we were children. I didn't need to see him all the time to know he was there.

Then in the last two years, as siblings on the threshold of old age, we've looked back together into our past. And we've become the only spectators, the only people who would care, watching our dad shrinking.

'Do you think it's possible to predict the future?' I say.

'Yes, I think I do,' he replies. 'But probably only the same way Dad did. Certainly not the way Mum did – or you might do, I don't know. Dad would have said time is just part of space. We don't yet know how to see forward in it, or travel forward in it. Other than by living, of course.'

'Dad's favourite book of all was about a time-travelling tattooist. *The Illustrated Man*, by Ray Bradbury. Not the choice of somebody who is only ever rational. It's about someone who meets a stranger with tattoos all over his body that move and predict the future. I think, when it came down to it, Dad had just as many fantastical notions as Mum did, he just expressed them differently.'

'Space science is really just sci-fi fantasy dressed up as physics,' my brother says. 'But if Dad thought he was about to die, he's more likely to have thought about the parallel with black holes than with some spooky made-up story, no matter how much he liked *The Illustrated Man*.'

'Why do you think so?'

'Well, only because that's what I'd think. There's an event horizon at the edge of a black hole, but you can't really see it. You can only see how things react to it. So, for a while, things seem normal. Everything's changing so gradually you aren't aware of it. Once you know it's there, you might think you're going to get away with it. Then you get closer, and sooner or later you realise it's pulling you in. Then you spaghettify—'

'You what?'

'Spaghettify – the fall is so steep it stretches you out, long and thin, like spaghetti.'

'Okay . . .'

'And according to general relativity, time slows down. Because of the bending effect of the gravitational field.'

'It might feel like a reprieve, then,' I say, 'if time is running slowly. Like you might have time to put things right and save yourself.'

'Unfortunately, though, as you go over the event horizon, the edge before you're in the black hole itself, then you'd know you've got no choices left. You must go in only one direction. You fall in and accelerate at phenomenal speed. That's when you might split into parallel selves, in different versions of space-time. Though you'd appear to be intact and motionless.'

'So, anybody watching would think you were fine,' I say.

'Quite. But you're heading straight for the singularity.'

'What's that like?'

'It's compressed matter,' my brother says. 'And at the same time, it's concentrated nothing, outside time.'

'You sound like a priest,' I say.

65

Friday, 26 September 1986, night
Michael takes down his old copy of *The Illustrated Man* and turns
it over in his hands. Then he opens it, a few pages in. 'He bared
his back,' he reads.

> *'See? There's no special design on my right shoulder
> blade, just a jumble.'*
> *'Yes.'*
> *'When I've been around a person long enough, that
> spot clouds over and fills in. If I'm with a woman, her
> picture comes there on my back, in an hour, and shows
> her whole life – how she'll live, how she'll die, what she'll
> look like when she's sixty. And if it's a man . . .'*

Michael touches the words on the page, which have begun to move.

> *'And if it's a man, an hour later his picture's here on
> my back. It shows him falling off a cliff. Or dying under
> a train . . .'*

Michael strokes his thumb across the book's edge to find the last
page, inside the soft back cover. As he opens the book again, his
face is bathed in bluish light, reflected from the full moon above

the scene inside. The Illustrated Man is lying there on the dusty ground, sleeping, with his head resting on a rounded stone. He is curled round like a child, barefoot and naked above the waist. The gentle sound of his breathing is synchronised with the rhythmic expansion and contraction of his body. Michael searches across the man's back for the empty space to find the void where the future might form.

As he watches, a patch of skin begins to crawl and catches his eye. A place on the man's shoulder blade, a little larger than a hand, is beginning to change. Gradually, the blur becomes more recognisable. At first it is a whirl of distortions, as if the face that's forming there is pressed up against a bullet glass window. Then the features are pulled taut by an invisible force into an awful grimace. Then they melt into each other like warm wax. As the image clears, Michael sees, unmistakeably, himself.

He shuts the book and throws it aside.

'No,' he says.

'No – not me. Not that. Not now.'

66

Friday, 26 September 1986, night
Michael watches himself walking back along the corridor from the study, empty handed. The passage rolls through 360 degrees, inverting him for a moment as he spirals into the living room.

He can see her there, but different this time. This time, she's sitting stiffly at the dining table.

'I couldn't find them. But never mind,' he says. 'Maybe there is something in what they're saying in the paper. Not all of it, of course. Or most of it. Maybe a little bit, round the edges.'

'They've libelled you, Michael,' she says steadily. Her mood has changed again. 'What exactly do you think we'll do, if you don't stop it from getting into all the papers? Can't you see? What on earth would we do?'

There's a noticeable acceleration, although he knows very well that he's standing perfectly still.

This is the only way, he thinks. There'll never be another opportunity like this, to finally make a clean breast of it.

'We've probably got enough money to just retire,' he says. 'We can just live here. Quietly. If we're careful.'

He turns to look at the perfect, pale room, sweeping his left hand around the space in a proprietorial gesture. His wedding ring slides along his finger then falls to the ground unnoticed with a gentle metallic sound, rolling away across the tiled floor.

This is going well, he thinks happily.

I think it's all going to be fine.

It's starting to sound quite hopeful, like there might be a future after all. He picks up the near-empty bottle and his empty glass and wanders out onto the terrace, then down the steps onto the lawn and towards the pool. A lizard senses the vibrations from the uneven impact of his shuffling feet on the stone flags and disappears into a crack in the parched ground.

Michael rests the bottle on a wooden sunlounger as he sits down heavily on another. He falls back, then rests the glass against his chest before closing his eyes. Very soon he's breathing in time with the rhythmic respiration of the pool filter.

We can just live here, quietly. In the house. And the garden.

A peaceful life. Maybe we'll – I don't know. Grow things.

Her voice goes off suddenly in his head, like an alarm.

'Grow things?' she shouts.

'For God's sake, Michael! Our lives, our careers, every bloody word we've ever written. There'll be literally nothing left!'

'I'm sure it won't be as bad as all that,' Michael says.

'Don't you think there'll be consequences, once you're nothing but a notorious fraud? And if people think you cheated them, why should they stop coming after us until they've taken every penny we have?'

On second thoughts, he might need to think that through, before bringing it up.

'If you believe for one second you can just walk away from all this and "grow things",' she demands, somewhere in his mind. 'Then frankly, Michael, I could kill you.'

At Victoria station, he's looking up at the departure board for the time of the next train to the airport.

'I wonder what's happening to me?' he says.

Dad, I think you're in a multiverse. You're still in London but you're at home in Spain as well. I think you're splitting apart.

67

'So, what's to be done?'

The disembodied voice starts up again at dawn, an unexpected intrusion, waking him suddenly from an uneasy dream. But at least she seems to have calmed down.

He can't immediately remember where he is. His eyelids remain closed against a sharp spasm that's beginning to pull against his temples. Twin images of a huge orange sun are printing themselves directly onto his eyeballs, through the thin skin.

It must be early, he thinks. But he can already feel his exposed chest and stomach burning. His mouth and throat are dry and rough with grit. He's wedged between the rigid armrests of a poolside bed with bare wooden slats digging into his flesh; there's an empty bottle overturned on the grass beside him.

When his eyes finally open and adjust to the blinding intensity of the light, his worst fear has not in fact been realised. She still isn't there. There's nobody there. He still has time. Although the optimism that carried him along during the previous evening appears to have evaporated.

He rolls out of the chair and takes off his clothes, leaving on just his boxer shorts. At the shaded corner of the pool, under the trees, he slides into the cool water and allows it to close over his head.

For a while, he floats around in the silence of the deep blue. Like the astronauts in that story. The story in *The Illustrated Man*.

What was it called?

'Kaleidoscope'?

His legs and feet hang weightless, his arms drift out idly from his sides.

She wouldn't believe it anyway, he thinks.

There's probably no point upsetting her any further.

He rehearses the homecoming scene once more, but this time from a safe distance. He's outside the lunar module now, carrying out a few routine repairs. If he isn't in the house then she'll come and find him in the garden. She'll still be smartly dressed from her meeting. Her outline crystallises then undulates among the clouds floating on the surface of the water. He closes his eyes again.

He imagines her walking purposefully now, along the mosaic-tiled edge towards the diving board. She steps up onto it with one stiletto-heeled foot, then the other. It bends a little under her weight, flexing with each step until she's standing suspended above him.

'They can't prove any of it anyway, can they?' she says, brightly. She kicks off her shoes and pulls her skirt up to her thighs, then she sits down on the end of the springboard with her stockinged feet dangling in mid-air.

'The so-called fake research. There's no real proof of what they're saying, is there? Not really. You just have to keep going, Michael.'

She points at him with a painted fingernail.

'If you just screw your courage to the sticking place, we can show that judge it's all just jealousy. It's all supposition and hearsay. And we won't let them get away with it. Not in a million years! Because when all's said and done, they're a bunch of jumped-up nobodies.'

She laughs, swinging her legs rhythmically so the board dances beneath her.

'But you're somebody, Michael.

'You're really somebody.

'You're a man with an unimpeachable reputation.'

The sound of her car in the driveway breaks his reverie and he opens his eyes.

'Ah yes, my unimpeachable reputation,' he says, floating onto his back.

It is recognisably his own voice, but from an unimaginable distance away.

68

'My unimpeachable reputation.'

The train is slowing down to stop at the airport. Inside the carriage, the other passengers are pulling bags from underneath the seats and from overhead racks, hauling out heavy suitcases and stacking them around the doors and in the aisles.

Do I have to get off now? he wonders.

Do I really have to go?

I don't think so, Dad. You think you're in Spain, anyway. If you really want to, you could just stay here instead.

He remains in his seat while there's a brief, noisy commotion, then the doors click shut again. The few remaining passengers melt away, leaving him alone.

But if I don't go back to Spain, what will I do?

It doesn't really matter what you do anymore, Dad. You're going to die anyway, whatever you do.

How will I die?

It's all so long ago. But I still don't really know. I just know you do. Maybe you kill yourself, with poison. Maybe somebody kills you or has you killed. Maybe you fall out of a spaceship and you burn up in the atmosphere.

Why would somebody kill me?

All kinds of reasons. You were about to lose all your money. And I think you knew things, about the business of drugs, about

252

the past. Things that some people might not want you to talk about in a public court case.

Perhaps I do. I don't know. I've forgotten. I think I will stay here, for now. Where do you think I should go?

You could just go home. To our home, I mean. Where we all used to live. When I was small.

As the train whistles and starts forward, he sings 'Home in Pasadena' quietly to himself,

'*Oh, you railway station.*
Oh, you Pullman train.
Here's my reservation for my destination,
Far beyond the Western plain'

I don't think I'd mind so much if I fell out of a spaceship, he thinks. Like in the story, in *The Illustrated Man*. Like 'Kaleidoscope'.

The house isn't far from the next station on the line, the one beyond the airport. The station with the white-painted ticket office, not far from the brook.

69

'Are you listening to me, Michael? I said you're a man with an unimpeachable reputation.'

Michael is weightless, drifting in happy circles like the spaceman he'd always wanted to be. He takes a deep breath, then he tells the whole story to a cloudless sky. About his fabricated self, starting from what he thought must be the beginning. About his boyhood, when he flew high over Lancashire every night in a spaceship, like the ones in *Astonishing Science Fiction*. About Isaac Asimov, H G Wells, Ray Bradbury and Arthur Clarke, and the books he could open at random, where each new page told him the story of his own destiny. About the strange upturn in his fortunes after Marion appeared, and after *The Incredible Shrinking Man*. About the SS *Carinthia*, about Pasadena, about the rockets and the nuclear lightshow. And the blue and red books. Why, in the end, he'd had no choice, other than to be the scientist he'd created. But who, admittedly, wasn't ever there.

'That's the truth. All of it,' he says.

'And in answer to your point, that they can't prove it. Maybe it's true they can't prove what I did. But they can prove what I am. The blue and red theses, wherever they are. When somebody finds them, they'll prove exactly what I am. And it's what I am that's the problem. I can see that now. If what happened at Deakin had been the first stupid thing I'd ever done, that would be one thing. But, in fact, it's probably going to be the last.'

The shadow of a figure cuts out the sun.
'Who are you talking to, Michael?'
This time, she's really there. Beside the pool.
'Oh. Nobody,' he says.

70

What can I do? Is there anything I can do now to make up for a terrible and empty life? If only I could do one good thing to make up for the meanness I collected all these years and didn't even know was in me! But there's no one here but myself, and how can you do good all alone? You can't. Tomorrow night I'll hit Earth's atmosphere. I'll burn, he thought, and be scattered in ashes all over the continental lands. I'll be put to use. Just a little bit, but ashes are ashes and they'll add to the land. He fell swiftly, like a bullet, like a pebble, like an iron weight, objective, objective all of the time now, not sad or happy or anything, but only wishing he could do a good thing now that everything was gone, a good thing for just himself to know about. When I hit the atmosphere, I'll burn like a meteor.

'I wonder,' he said, 'if anyone'll see me?'

'Kaleidoscope' by Ray Bradbury, from *The Illustrated Man*

71

You don't really fall out of a spaceship and burn up in the atmosphere – at least, I don't think so.

I thought that wouldn't happen, at least not in this universe. Quite a lot of other things would have to be different for that Me, in that reality. I know there's something coming, though. It's on the shoulder of the Illustrated Man.

The truth is, I get a letter from your wife. She'll tell me soon you've started vomiting blood.

When? I mean, how long will it be, before she'll tell you?

The letter arrives in the ordinary overland post, so maybe a week after it happens, maybe more. Sometime in early November.

That does sound like poison, doesn't it? On the face of it. An acute toxic event. Strychnine maybe? I hope it isn't paraquat.

Somebody will take you to a hospital in Torremolinos but I don't know who. Your wife will visit you the following morning.

Then what?

Then. Then, I'm not telling you anymore. I'm sorry. There's nothing more I can say.

Nothing can come of nothing, you know that. Speak again.

Oh, Dad, you'll be alone, in a ward full of strangers. Crawling naked on the floor. Hiding under a bed, wrapped in a dirty sheet. And you'll scream like a frightened child.

So, I'm going to be mad, then. Soon I'll be a blanket-loined Bedlam beggar.

You'll see demons, Dad. You'll have visions . . .

Poison again. Renal failure, perhaps. So, tell me. What did you do?

What did I do? What could I do? I couldn't do anything. I did nothing.

Nothing? Why still nothing?

I'm so sorry, Dad. But I didn't know what to do. I send a telegram to your wife. I believe you're still alive when I do.

I can't predict how it will end. In any event, I don't.

The next day, she calls me from somewhere. That's when she tells me you're dead. She says your body has already gone. There's no point trying to see you, because you aren't there.

Well, I suppose if there isn't anything to do, then the only thing you could do is nothing. There's no need to be sorry about that. I suppose it's just what happens.

72

The telegram, then the phone call, then nothing. Then the third part of Dennis Potter's drama *The Singing Detective*, called 'Lovely Days', was on television for the first time on 30 November 1986, two days after I got the news my dad was dead.

'Lovely Days' begins at a railway station, where there are two people, but only one of them is leaving. When a whistle sounds, the engine starts to move. A father is standing on the edge of the platform with his arm raised, waving goodbye. A child departs, on a slowly moving train. The father walks along the platform, as if to be close to the child for as long as he can, but the train disappears and is gone. The singing detective of the child's imagination is on a stage with a dance band in a crowded night club: he sings 'Paper Doll', a song about the pain of lost love. As he sings, he raises his arm, waving back to his dad, even though he was left behind long ago, in the distant past. The sound of the train rises above the anxious pulse of heart monitors in a hospital ward, where a sick man is going mad, tormented by bizarre hallucinations. When the father appears again on the platform, he is mouthing the words of 'Paper Doll' alone in the rain, to himself.

It seemed to be a condensed and inverted interpretation of a scene I'd been in myself two months before. A parallel reality, another road to another kind of ending, with a station platform, a final train journey, a father and a child, and a deranged man in a hospital ward. One of us had been left behind on the platform, though in this other version of reality it would have been my dad, not me. The living world had been about to pull away without him, after all. Two days before I watched this scene, he had become an increasingly distant, solitary figure, waving goodbye at a station.

For a long time after the phone call, I couldn't hold the two ideas – my dad and my dad being dead – simultaneously in my mind. They were separate parts of a binary image, one left, one right; each of them on their own was a realistic but partial transparency. But when I moved them together and held them one over the other, the combined picture was lost, forming a meaningless blur. Apart again, the images returned to clarity.

This one is him. This one is him too, only dead.

Maybe they'll never fit together because they're from two different realities. These two versions of him were never intended to make one complete whole.

Because there'll always be some other place again, in space or in time, where he's still there.

73

Friday, 26 September 1986, evening
Michael sits on the airport train considering the inevitable fate of the man who might now be telling the truth to his wife at Villa Valencia.

This is a grim future, he thinks. But even if this prophecy were true, surely it's nothing more than my daughter's story. It's about her, not me. It doesn't have to be my future at all. 'The Illustrated Man' is just a story too, by Ray Bradbury. In space and time, nothing is set in stone.

What if, with this consciousness I have, with this insight I've been given, I decide never to go back to Spain? Then I won't be there to bleed out on an Andalucian hillside and I won't be there in a Torremolinos hospital to die. Surely, now that I know, I have the right to choose another life before that happens? I can take myself in a completely different direction. I've done that before, many times.

There must have been a different route I could have taken, further back on the path, one that leads to an altogether better ending.

But to find it, I need to take a few steps back in time.

By chance – or is it chance? – I'm almost at the old house, the one beside the brook.

❖ ❖ ❖

Michael is alone in the carriage as the train brakes gently and comes to a stop. The station slides into view again, this time out of the darkness. Flickering illuminated shapes crisscross the ticket office at odd angles, forming a collection of facades, lines and surfaces, without structure or substance. The place is empty, as it had been before, and unmanned.

He opens the carriage door and steps down onto the grey, light-washed platform, then closes the door behind him.

The train moves away and very soon it's gone. He watches the rear light as it disappears into the distance, and then he walks to the end of the platform and over the metal bridge. He goes through a familiar gate and down the curving slope in the direction of the brook. A warmer glow spreads down the steps and into the underpass from orange bulkhead safety lights. He's aware of the call and echo from his hard-soled shoes, and the quiet counterpoint of dripping water. His shoes begin to move loosely on his feet and feel heavier than they were before. His heels tread mud into the sagging turnups of his trousers. His jacket won't stay on his shoulders and no longer seems to fit. After a while, he stops tugging it back and lets it fall behind him, onto the wet concrete.

As he emerges into the night, he can see that the mist has cleared from the surrounding fields. The ribbon of longer grass and rushes following the line of the brook is now an undifferentiated mass of deep black, seen against the lighter, undulating greys of the empty land around it. He remembers it all. Just over the hill is the house, his house, and further on is Schering. His house. His study, where his books and papers used to be. Where he'll have time to begin again.

He slides down the muddy bank on his feet and hands, then starts to make his way along the ditch, slipping here and there on wet grass as he inches forward, unseeing.

The world of the brook grows taller around him as his shoes sink deeply into the soft silt. He tries to steady himself but the mud and weeds suck hard on his feet. He falls sideways against the bank. He reaches up to grasp the dead stalks of bullrushes, freeing ghostly clouds from the dry pods into the cold night air. As he pulls himself free, his shoes stay still and his feet slide easily from them, past their tightly knotted laces. His silk socks are thin and wet, and he steps on them so they slide easily away, like shedding skin.

His bare toes reach and feel around under the water to find a foothold each time he takes a step. He's alive to all the sensations that can keep him upright and moving, and to the sound of his own breathing. From time to time, something splashes unseen in the shallow water. A toad, perhaps. But he doesn't feel afraid.

Soon he makes out a shape and a glow not far in front of him, as he moves through the field.

The house is just as he remembered. It's alone in its space, in a wide garden edged on either side by sycamore trees. Its three flat roofs gave it a symmetrical outline, with single-storey sections extending out to either side of a larger living space. It's mostly glass, and slightly lifted from its natural foundations on concealed pillars. Now, at night, it seems to hover like a spaceship landing on a suburban lawn.

The interior lights flick on, filling the huge windows with an intense brightness. Parabolic beams project across the patio and onto the grass, falling just short of where he is standing. Looking up out of the darkness, he can see everything inside, as if the front of the doll's house has swung open. It's still painted perfect white.

Nothing has changed, he thinks. Maybe I haven't changed. Maybe no time has passed at all.

The far end of the garden falls away towards the brook with no fence to separate them. He is standing in a thin stream of shallow, moving water, although he is no longer aware that his feet are numb with cold. His hands are bleeding from scores of tiny cuts made by the sharp blades of the rushes. He rubs away the blood and dirt on the tails of his shirt, then he scrambles up the bank and lies down on his stomach with his face resting on his folded arms.

Inside the pure white living room, a woman appears and dances weightlessly round and round in an elliptical pattern, carrying a small child in her arms. As she floats to the window, he can see she is barefoot and that her hair is close cropped, like a boy. A man appears, drifting close enough to kiss her, then he lifts the child from her, holding her up high, whirling her round. He is in shirtsleeves, his tie hanging loose, his suit jacket abandoned somewhere else, maybe on the hall stand where Michael used to leave his own. The woman seems to pass through an unseen valve, materialising a moment later in the kitchen. The child floats up to stroke the man's cheek with her hand. He puts his hand over hers and she laughs as he reaches out to kiss her.

The man settles the girl into the crook of his arm as he points upwards towards something outside, in the sky. She can see it too and, in her delight, she stretches out her own small hands towards it. He walks outside, until he's close enough to Michael to touch him. Still holding his daughter, talking softly to her.

'I wonder,' Michael says aloud, 'if anyone can see me?'

They stand beside him unaware, watching the meteor burning brightly as it falls.

Objective, objective all the time now, Michael thinks. Not sad or happy or anything. He knows he's falling swiftly: like a bullet, like a pebble, like an iron weight.

If only I could do one good thing, he thinks. Now that everything is gone.

But he knows in that moment that it's hopeless to think it could ever have been any other way. If it were on a hospital floor, or in a muddy ditch, under a train, or falling from the sky, it really makes no difference.

And Michael starts to cry, as the little girl makes a wish.

74

'When life is over,' Hollis thinks to himself as he falls towards the Earth, 'it is like a flicker of bright film.' 'An instant on the screen' is all it ever could have been.

In the Ray Bradbury story 'Kaleidoscope', the men make small talk on their helmet radios as each floats in a different direction to a particular and certain fate. Hollis is drawn inexorably into the Earth's atmosphere, where he catches fire and is reduced to powder. Wood spins away towards the moon. Stone finds himself suddenly surrounded by a cluster of dancing asteroids and is carried along in its brightness to the farthest edge of the solar system.

Drifting alone in space, Hollis believes that the moment of dying is always the same, no matter where it might be or how sudden or surprising the cause. And that the end will come too quickly and too soon. Life shrinks to a vanishing point, 'all of its prejudices and passions condensed and illumined for an instant on space', as everything that seemed to matter very much ceases to matter at all.

My dad's last flicker of bright film is still in an inaccessible vault at the British Film Institute, in a safe deposit box with a lost key. If the time comes when all that's hidden is made manifest, even by the English courts and the BFI, maybe I'll sit in an empty movie theatre as the lights go down, while the projectionist forces the lock, then winds through to find that unseen nine minutes of magnetic tape. Threading it onto the spool, then lighting the lamp and letting it run. Film can bring back the dead, but only in this case for one last 540 seconds. It's a wonder of our age, all the same, if my dad were to be reanimated, twenty feet tall, now I'm so much older than him then, older than he ever was. So many decades ago, when his star was at its brightest. And then I think I should let him finally melt away.

Hollis also foresaw a last picture show taking place on his incendiary fall from a starry sky. For him, it was a kaleidoscope of tiny fragments from his past, the life that is often said to flash before the eyes of the dying. But: 'before you could cry out "there was a happy day, there a bad one, there an evil face, there a good one", the film burned to a cinder and the screen went dark.'

75

Sometime after my brother and I had left home, my mother opened a small shop where she sold crystals and silver jewellery, and sometimes dispensed miracle cures and mystical advice. She lived for long enough to see my brother and me find a firm foot-hold in the adult world, and she knew and loved all three of her grandchildren. But as time went on, vascular dementia, which was probably a consequence of the hypercalcaemia that overshadowed her late twenties and thirties, magnified some of her existing qual-ities in a way that made her increasingly difficult to negotiate with or care for. The last couple of years were very frustrating for her because she continued to believe there was a better life somewhere else that she was being deliberately prevented from having, prob-ably by me. When she died, my brother and I agreed to wait a little while before marking the fact that she'd gone, so we could gather our thoughts. In the meantime, she was cremated, unobserved.

Two months later, in late August 2015, my mother's ashes were interred in the rose garden of the church in the village that became her adopted home, and mine. The church has stained glass Pre-Raphaelite angels with bias-cut satin celestial garments and the faces of poets. People came to say goodbye from the many different lives she'd lived: the painters and sculptors, the pattern-cutters, seamstresses and stylists, the local friends, the customers and shop staff, the jazz crowd she danced with on Sunday afternoons, the extended family. We read nonsense verse by Spike Milligan, Rudyard Kipling's 'The Crab that Played with Sea', and the Book of Jonah. We listened to Mahalia Jackson's 'Move On Up a Little Higher'. The grandchildren played 'Tiger Rag' on a variety of instruments, celebrating the frantic bedtime tiger hunts she'd created when they were still small enough to believe.

My partner played the ukulele and sang her song for her, one last time. I think she'd only ever been truly happy in the place and time that was Pasadena, when she'd been the Liverpool factory girl who fled and found herself in southern California, as if by magic. With a successful Space-Age husband and a new baby son, even she couldn't believe her luck.

So, I think I'll be on my way,
To that dreamland from yesterday;
Tell the mailman I'm going to stay
Where grass is greener.
I'll settle down in that pretty town
That's the place where I'll be found,
There'll be a house and a car around, and the sunshine
on my door.
Beneath the palms, there beneath those palms,
In someone's arms.
At last, I'm home
In Pasadena town.

By the end, my dad's world, which he had tried to make the whole world, had shrunk until it was vanishingly small. He'd reached for the stars and had fallen very far. It's likely my dad took some secrets with him when he died, and if he'd lived, he would have implicated others in his deceptions. Whatever he did that led to the 1986 research scandal, it's very unlikely he did it alone.

My dad never met any of his grandchildren. He didn't see my nieces grow into funny, warm and beautiful young women, and natural mathematicians like their father. He didn't meet my son, or the man my son fell in love with, who we all then fell in love with too.

My mother never entirely gave up hope: she always believed there was still a chance of reconciliation, although redemption might have been a better word for it. As the years passed, her feelings had to adapt to impossibility, to the paradox of loving a man so changed he could no longer be seen.

But to her, like Scott was to Louise, he would never be nothing.

As far as I know, my dad was buried on 28 November 1986, within a few hours of his death. I heard about it after it had happened and the only mourner present was his wife, a doctor and fertility specialist who had co-authored several of his later publications. He had to be buried immediately because it was a Friday, and I believe that's what happens in the south of Spain. According to the certificate, he was pronounced dead by seven o'clock and the paperwork was completed by ten o'clock that morning. Whatever arrangements there were, they must have been made very quickly. The cause of his death is not recorded.

My dad's widow sold up quickly and moved on, back to England, where within a few years she'd married again. Life goes on, after all. If you walk around any graveyard, you will always see one or two memorials with a space left blank for a second guest, the one who decided in the end that they would rather sleep somewhere else. Time passes and we are all entitled to change our minds.

By the time of his death, there were very few people left apart from his wife who might have thought of my dad with any fondness. As far as I know, there was only my brother, myself and, in her bruised and compromised way, my mother. To the three of us, his death only added another layer to his already well-established absence. He was already so far away, anyway.

These days, I hardly ever think about the possibility, remote though it is, that in 1986 he didn't die at all. I stopped listening for an unexpected knock at the door quite a few years ago. Or wondering if he could have led another life somewhere, as someone else. Imagined alternatives made it difficult at the time to think of my dad's death as just another ordinary tragedy, of an ordinary father who died too young, being mourned by his children. As is sometimes the way.

When I say my dad was buried, that isn't strictly true. He wasn't interred, he was immured. His body was inserted into a small compartment in a burial wall at the large municipal cemetery in Torremolinos, then the opening was sealed shut with a stone. I have seen a photograph of it but I confess I've never had the desire to visit.

Even if I had, I'm told that this way of dealing with a corpse above the ground is time limited by licence, twenty years being quite long enough for many. If the licence isn't renewed, then the tomb is emptied and swept clean of whatever remains inside. The climate is, in this sense, ideal, as all that's usually needed is a long-handled brush. Empty tombs are left open for a while, so the wind can blow through and put the last of any dust to good use. Then the vacant space can be rented again, by somebody else.

So, to be honest, he probably isn't there anyway.

POSTSCRIPT

The striking-out of the Primodos case in 2023 ended all related clinical negligence claims against Bayer Schering and claims for regulatory failures by the UK government. Those people who are still living with disabilities that they believe were caused pre-birth by Primodos, an unnecessary and now unlicensable pharmacological product, are all around retirement age. Marie Lyon was awarded the British Empire Medal in the King's Honours List in 2024, in recognition of her continuing work as a campaigner on behalf of the victims of hormone pregnancy tests.

Journalist Jason Farrell may make a second film for Sky News about the Primodos scandal, following on from the success of *Primodos: A Bitter Pill*. It is likely to focus on whether the conclusions of the Expert Working Group were fatally flawed.

Pressure within the British Parliament from a cross-party group of MPs is increasing. The Cumberlege recommendations are being implemented for people injured by pelvic mesh and sodium valproate.

But nothing at all has been done about Baroness Cumberlege's recommended compensation scheme for people who suffered avoidable harm from the use of Primodos.

ACKNOWLEDGEMENTS

I would not have written this story at all if it hadn't been for the first Bridport Prize memoir competition. I decided to put down the first 8,000 words and send them in as a 59th birthday present to myself, on 30 September 2022. Everyone in the Bridport Prize process was unfailingly kind and helpful, and winning the competition was a truly overwhelming experience. I'm profoundly grateful to the panel of judges, led by bestselling memoirist and author Cathy Rentzenbrink. The prize package included editorial feedback from Anna South, which helped me begin the next stage of the journey.

I'm very grateful to my agents Euan Thorneycroft and Florence Rees at A.M. Heath for being able to see my story's potential. Their support and guidance over the following year helped turn a 30,000-word competition entry into a full-length manuscript. My publishers, Sarah Braybrooke and Ellie Carr at Ithaka Press, and my editor Liz Marvin, each provided their own invaluable inspirations and insights. During the edit, I gave Liz my knitting and she kindly showed me the best way to stitch it together, then turned it the right way out for me.

Thank you to Marie Lyon BEM, the chair of the Association for Children Damaged by Hormone Pregnancy Tests (ACDHPT) for her knowledge, her commitment, her enthusiasm and her friendship. Jason Farrell at Sky News has been committed to the

Primodos story for over a decade, and I thank him for the conversations we've had that have helped me to understand some of its complexities. Before his sad death in February 2024, I was able to express my gratitude to Professor Barrie Kitto, and once again I send my condolences to Binnie.

I'm indebted to the many archivists who have helped me find the information I needed, despite the passing of several decades; particularly to those at Cornell, Wellington and the University of the Arts in London. My brother, Dr Andrew Briggs, has been consistently himself, which is a blessing to me. Not for the first time, he has tolerated a manifestation of his younger sister's unhealthy curiosity without complaint. Thanks to my great friend Dr Sandra Virgo, who explains statistics better than anyone else I know. And to the women who helped me think it all through, in the sea and out of it, summer and winter, twice around: not only, but particularly, Alice, George, and Jude.

My partner, Mike Mole, helped in too many ways to list them all, from plot development and literary insights to proofreading and lost document recovery. My aunt, Bebe, and my cousins, Daniela and Steven, provided kind words of encouragement as this curious footnote in their own lives was being written. My son James Buck and his partner Luke Brooks were always there when they were most needed and never doubted that this story would one day become a book.

SELECTED BIBLIOGRAPHY

Books, journals and websites

Studies of the Biochemistry of Biotin and its Analogues. Cornell University *MSc*, M H Briggs, 1958

Handbook of Philosophy, M H Briggs, Philosophical Library Inc. New York, 1959

Studies on the Biochemistry of Biotin and its Analogues, M H Briggs, 1959

The Chemistry and Metabolism of Drugs and Toxins: An Introduction to Xenobiochemistry, M H Briggs & M Briggs, 1974

Current Aspects of Exobiology, Eds: G Mamikunian & M H Briggs, 1965

Reflections of a Whistle-Blower, Jim Rossiter, 1992

'De omnibus rebus et de quibusdam aliis: Review of "Current Aspects of Exobiology"', Carl Sagan, *Quarterly Review of Biology* vol. 41 no.4, 1966

The Anatomy of a Fraud: Symmetry and Dance, Robert Trivers, Brian G Palestis, Darine Zaatari, 2009

'Who's Afraid of Peer Review?', John Bohannon, article in *Science* magazine, 2013

Are We Alone?, The Stanley Kubrick Extraterrestrial-Intelligence Interviews, edited Anthony Frewin, 2005

Humans to Mars, Fifty Years of Mission Planning 1950–2000, David S Portree, NASA History Division, 2001

Eyes on the Red Planet: Human Mars Mission Planning 1952–1970, Anne M Platoff, UC Santa Barbara, 2001

'Obituary of Frederick C Ordway', *New York Times*, 13 July 2013

Jet Propulsion Laboratory History, NASA JPL website, https://www.jpl.nasa.gov/who-we-are/history

'Going Nuclear Over the Pacific', Gilbert King, *Smithsonian*, 2012

The Time Machine, H G Wells, 1895

The War of the Worlds, H G Wells, 1898

There Will Come Soft Rains, Ray Bradbury, 1950

'The Talking Stone', Isaac Asimov, 1955

The Light of Other Days, Arthur C Clarke & Stephen Baxter, 2000

'Kaleidoscope' from *The Illustrated Man*, Ray Bradbury, 1951

'There Will Come Soft Rains', Sara Teasdale, 1918

Social Problems of the North, Charles Edward Bellyse Russell, 1913

The Time That Is Left, Giorgio Agamben, University of Verona, 2002

Bleak House, Charles Dickens, 1853

Film, TV and Music

Catch Me If You Can, dir. Steven Spielberg, Dreamworks Pictures, 2002

2001: A Space Odyssey, dir. Stanley Kubrick, Metro-Goldwyn-Mayer, 1968

Quatermass and the Pit, BBC Television, 1958

The Singing Detective, Dennis Potter, BBC Television, 1986

The Incredible Shrinking Man, screenplay by Richard Matheson & Richard Alan Simmons, Universal Pictures, 1957

Rollerball, screenplay by William Harrison, dir. Norman Jewison, United Artists, 1975

'Home in Pasadena', music by Harry Warren, lyrics by Grant Clarke and Edgar Leslie, 1923

Corsham Tunnels/Burlington Bunker

The Timeline of Britain's Most Secret Bunker, Burlington, Higgypop https://www.higgypop.com/news/burlington-bunker, 2010

Corsham Tunnels – A Brief History, ISS (Information Systems & Services), Ministry of Defence, 2016

MOD Corsham Wiltshire Values Study, English Heritage/Oxford Archaeology, 2010

'Civil Defence Policy in Cold War Britain 1945–68', Matthew Grant, Queen Mary, University of London (PhD)

Struggle for Survival, Steve Fox, Subterranea Britannica, https://www.subbrit.org.uk/features/struggle-for-survival

Wiltshire's Underground City, BBC Wiltshire website, https://www.bbc.co.uk/wiltshire/underground_city, 2014

Schering AG/Primodos/Jenapharm

Wilson & Others v Bayer Pharma AG & Others, [2023] EWHC 1282 (KB), Yip, J, judgment, 2023

'The Bogus Work of Professor Briggs', Brian Deer, *Sunday Times* 1986

The Briggs Affair Parts 1–3, Deakin University Library Blog, 2022

First Do No Harm, Baroness Cumberlege, 2020

Schering AG – Company Profile, Information, Business Description, History, Background Information on Schering AG, ReferenceForBusiness.com,

The role of the State Security Service (Stasi) in the context of international clinical trials conducted by western pharmaceutical companies in Eastern Germany (1961–1990), National Library of Medicine, Ed: Lorenz von Seidlein, 2018

Bitter Pill: Primodos, Sky News documentary, 2017

A Bitter Pill: Primodos – The Forgotten Thalidomide, UK All-Party Parliamentary Group for Hormone Pregnancy Tests, 2024

'Hormonal doping and androgenization of athletes: a secret program of the German Democratic Republic government', Werne W Franke & Brigitte Berendonk, *Clinical Chemistry,* vol. 43 iss. 7, 1997